"As pharmaceutical companies are starting to spend big on 'electroceutical' research, Dr. Corradino reminds us that much of this work has already been done. Building upon years of experience would be a wise move in that quest, and this book offers an all-important brick in the understanding of bioelectric medicine. Dr. Corradino provides real and clear teachings based in his own research and clinical practice to benefit both the Eastern and Western physician. Stay ahead of the game—read this book."

—*Dr. Laura Kelly, author of* The Healthy Bones
Nutrition Plan and Cookbook

"Dr. Corradino's development of the Neuropuncture system is cutting-edge acupuncture. As our profession advances and continues to become more mainstream, this content is invaluable to both new and seasoned acupuncturists. Dr. Corradino does a great job explaining the evidence-based neurophysiological mechanisms of acupuncture and presents highly effective treatment protocols. *Neuropuncture* is a deep dive into the world of modern biomedical acupuncture. I am extremely grateful for this much-needed contribution to our profession."

—*Andy Rosenfarb, N.D., L.Ac., Doctor of Naturopathic Medicine,
Board Certified in Acupuncture and Chinese Herbal Medicine*

T0173660

of related interest

The Fundamentals of Acupuncture
Nigel Ching
Foreword by Charles Buck
ISBN 978 1 84819 313 0
eISBN 978 0 85701 266 1

Psycho-Emotional Pain and the Eight Extraordinary Vessels
Yvonne R. Farrell, DAOM, L.AC.
ISBN 978 1 84819 292 8
eISBN 978 0 85701 239 5

Cosmetic Acupuncture, Second Edition
A Traditional Chinese Medicine Approach to
Cosmetic and Dermatological Problems
Radha Thambirajah
ISBN 978 1 84819 267 6
eISBN 978 0 85701 215 9

Neuropuncture

A Clinical Handbook of Neuroscience Acupuncture
Second Edition

Michael D. Corradino
Foreword by Giovanni Maciocia

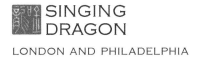

SINGING
DRAGON

LONDON AND PHILADELPHIA

First edition published in 2012 by Michael D. Corradino
This second edition first published in 2017
by Singing Dragon
an imprint of Jessica Kingsley Publishers
73 Collier Street
London N1 9BE, UK
and
400 Market Street, Suite 400
Philadelphia, PA 19106, USA

www.singingdragon.com

Library of Congress Cataloging in Publication Data
Title: Neuropuncture : a clinical handbook of neuroscience acupuncture /
    Michael Corradino.
Description: Second edition. | London ; Philadelphia : Jessica Kingsley
    Publishers, 2017. | Includes bibliographical references.
Identifiers: LCCN 2016042884 (print) | LCCN 2016044233 (ebook) | ISBN
    9781848193314 (alk. paper) | ISBN 9780857012876 (ebook)
Subjects: | MESH: Acupuncture Therapy--methods | Nervous System Physiological
    Phenomena
Classification: LCC RM184 (print) | LCC RM184 (ebook) | NLM WB 369 | DDC
    615.8/92--dc23

British Library Cataloguing in Publication Data
A CIP catalogue record for this book is available from the British Library

ISBN 978 1 84819 331 4
eISBN 978 0 85701 287 6

Printed and bound in Great Britain

Contents

Foreword to the First Edition

Acupuncture is a very rich tradition characterized by many different styles, theories, and approaches, inspired by the medicine of different countries such as China, Vietnam, Japan, and Korea, and now, Western countries. It is a powerful medicine that has proved its value over thousands of years starting in China and now practiced literally all over the world.

There are many ways of practicing acupuncture: far from detracting from it, this diversity enriches it. If we see this diversity from a "traditional" and, I would say, Daoist perspective, we can accept it and embrace it. Seen from a "scientific" perspective, this diversity poses a problem. How can we treat the same person and the same problem in so many different ways, with all of them effective? Of course we can: life is fluid and rich, and acupuncture is a therapy that treats the person addressing the whole person through the channels. The ancient Chinese word for "body" (that the channels treat) is shen [身]. Although often translated as "body," it is more than the body, and it could be said to be the "self," or the "person." Interestingly, the word shen for "body" has the same sound as the word shen for "mind" and "spirit."

In the modern, Western world, we have a new diversity of acupuncture practice: "traditional" versus "scientific." I use the quotation marks around those two words intentionally as they are words that are open to interpretation and misunderstanding. It would be difficult to define what "traditional" acupuncture is: is the one from the Han dynasty more traditional than the styles practiced much later in the Qing dynasty? Is Japanese acupuncture more "traditional" than Chinese because it tends to follow the more ancient classics? Is an acupuncturist who uses laser for the stimulation of points not "traditional"?

The word "scientific" is also open to interpretation. Is "scientific" acupuncture one that dismisses the concept of channels altogether in favor of nerves as an explanation of how acupuncture works? Or is it a type of acupuncture whose practitioners use only protocols deriving from published studies?

Unfortunately, the two camps of "traditional" and "scientific" acupuncture do not seem to meet at all. For example, Dr. Felix Mann says in his book *Reinventing Acupuncture: A New Concept of Ancient Medicine*: "The traditional acupuncture points are no more real than the black spots a drunkard sees in front of his eyes" (Mann, 2000, p.14). He also says: "The meridians of acupuncture are no more real than the meridians of geography. If someone were to get a spade and try to dig up the Greenwich meridian, he might end up in a lunatic asylum. Perhaps the same fate should await those doctors who believe in [acupuncture] meridians" (Mann, 2000, p.31).

White and Campbell (2005) say in the *British Medical Journal Online*:

> Traditional Chinese medicine includes a number of concepts that are contrary to the current prevailing understanding of anatomy and physiology. One is the whole idea of "meridians." Another is the very basis of diagnosis and treatment: that a particular set of points can be chosen to treat "Liver fire rising" and a different set of points chosen to treat "Dampness in the Spleen." This belief system requires the suspension of disbelief by many Western practitioners and patients, and raises questions about the use of belief in medicine, credulity, and patient autonomy.

They also say:

> There is an alternative theoretical model that provides a solution to the "paradox" of RCT results in acupuncture: that the needles stimulate nerves, not meridians and points. Therefore, for many conditions, the needle can be inserted almost anywhere within the

relevant spinal segment: it is the skin or muscle penetration that is sufficient. (White & Campbell, 2005)

It is regrettable that there should be such a contrast between "traditional" and "scientific" acupuncture, a contrast that is totally unnecessary. I would count myself among those who practice "traditional" acupuncture and yet I do realize and accept that acupuncture must work through the nervous system as well as channels. Apart from the fact, of course, that Traditional Chinese Medicine is indeed "scientific" but not according to the paradigm of modern biomedicine.

It is interesting that similar contrasts existed also in ancient China although not couched in terms of "traditional" versus "scientific." In ancient China, shamans practiced their art, consisting in ridding the body and mind of evil spirits through incantations. Before the Warring States Period (476–221 BC), shamanism was the main form of healing. From the Warring States onwards, healing began to be practiced by acupuncturists and herbalists. However, shamanism continued to be practiced alongside acupuncture and herbal medicine. We could compare the shamans to today's "traditional acupuncturists," and the ancient acupuncturists themselves to today's advocates of "scientific" acupuncture.

There were times in ancient China when some provincial governors tried to suppress the practice of shamanism in favor of the acupuncture practiced according to the principles of Yin Yang and the Five Elements. Interestingly, during the Song dynasty (AD 960–1279), Xia Song, Prefect of Hongzhou, took action against more than 1900 shamans in his jurisdiction. He had their shrines destroyed and forced them to "change occupation and apply themselves to the practice of acumoxa, prescription and pulse-taking" (Hindrichs & Barnes, 2013, p.109).

However, such intolerance is rare in ancient China, and the much more prevalent attitude was to simply accept both shamanism and acupuncture and indeed combine and integrate the two. For example, during the Tang dynasty (AD 618–907), the Imperial Medical College had a Department of Incantations and the great doctor Sun Si Miao (AD 581–682) made no difference between the beneficial effects of medical decoctions, acupuncture, incantations, and talismans (Hindrichs & Barnes, 2013).

Dr. Corradino's book follows firmly in Sun Si Miao's tradition of tolerance and integration, i.e. the integration between traditional acupuncture and one that takes the nervous system into account. Indeed, even for this reason only, Dr. Corradino's book is an important milestone in the development of acupuncture and of integrative medicine. No other book on acupuncture integrates seamlessly the traditional knowledge of channels and points with the nervous system. For example, Dr. Corradino points out that "if we align a chart of the Yin meridians with a chart of the upper arm nerve pathways, they are almost identical."

Dr. Corradino has huge clinical experience in the treatment of pain, with his system integrating acupuncture according to channels and according to nerves. There is no contradiction between the two and its practice does not diminish or invalidate "traditional acupuncture" at all.

In Chapter 4, Dr. Corradino discusses a fascinating review of the neural and humoral mechanisms of acupuncture but he integrates it with the traditional view of channels and quotations from the *Nei Jing*. In the fascinating Chapter 6, he reviews major points, integrating the classical indications with those from neural anatomy.

I believe that Dr. Corradino's book is a major contribution to the integration of acupuncture in modern biomedicine, without acupuncture "losing its soul," and one that is essential to the treatment of pain in particular.

Giovanni Maciocia
Santa Barbara, 2013

Acknowledgments

I would like to extend an enormous thank you to my family for their continued support. To John Hubacher with Pantheon research, the team of IAREA, Duong Ha, James Dunn, Laura Kelly, Lorne Brown with PROD Seminars, "Don Gio"—Giovanni Maciocia—and always and forever mia bambina, Ana Gancheva and AG Creative Solutions. I would also like to thank Singing Dragon for taking on this project with me. Without them this would not be able to reach the masses as intended.

About the Author

Dr. Michael Corradino graduated from Pacific College of Oriental Medicine, Cum Laude, in 1995 with a Masters in Traditional Oriental Medicine (MTOM). He has been in the field of Integrated Chinese Medicine since his graduation (20+ years). His mission in life is to expose quality Integrative Traditional Chinese Medicine (TCM) to as many people as possible in his lifetime, in order to present an effective, quality option for health care, while aiding the integration of Eastern, Western, and Natural medicine. While on the east coast, Dr. Corradino ran a very successful acupuncture treatment company in New York, as well as owning an acupuncture medical billing company. He relinquished his acupuncture contracts and relocated to San Diego in 2004 to complete his Doctorate in Acupuncture and Oriental Medicine (DAOM) in an effort to further enrich and deepen his understanding of TCM. It was at this time that he began to have deeper questions about the actual physiological mechanisms of acupuncture and began to research neurophysiology to investigate acupuncture in the area of neuroscience.

Dr. Corradino has been an educator for over a decade, teaching at Master and Doctoral levels. He has lectured at various professional institutions including UC Irvine School of Medicine, multiple professional Oriental and Acupuncture conferences, the Pacific Symposium, the San Diego Art Institute, and San Diego State University. He has been a guest on KUSI San Diego live morning news, had a health slot on the CS Keys sports talk show with *On the Mic with Dr. Mike*, presents continuing education unit (CEU)-accredited workshops on the theory and clinical applications of "Neuropuncture," an acupuncture system based on neuroscience, and more. He is also the resident practitioner and weekly speaker for the elite Golden Door Spa and Retreat, located in Southern California. Here he presents every week on several topics, all involving Chinese medicine. He has been featured on their special Speaker Series and is in the process of developing and launching a product line integrating Traditional Chinese herbal medicine with nutraceuticals into transdermal patches.

Dr. Corradino was one of the first DAOM graduates in the USA. This postgraduate doctorate is a two-and-a-half-year integrated clinical doctorate in TCM, which includes, but is not limited to, the study of the five main Chinese medical classics, Chinese medical language, advanced areas of specialty (neuromuscular), an integrated clinical internship, and a Capstone proposal in which Dr. Corradino ran a successful clinical Electro-Acupuncture trial on sciatica due to intervertebral disc herniation. He has also studied medicine under five highly renowned and experienced doctors at two hospitals and one medical school in China, completing the first "Five Masters' TCM Tour Program" in 2007.

Currently Dr. Corradino has two private practices in Southern California. As mentioned above, the first is the elite Golden Door Spa and Retreat. He also has a general practice, focusing on pain management, which is located inside Pain Care San Diego, an integrated pain center. He treats patients with a wide range of conditions as he focuses on applying neuroscience to every possible scenario in order to test its effectiveness across the board in all medical cases. His clinical interests include pain management, sports medicine, neurology, addiction medicine and pharmaceutical drug cessation treatments, neuromuscular conditions, general internal medicine such as cardiology and endocrinology, psychiatry, and general wellbeing/longevity.

Applying neurophysiology techniques to acupuncture and various types of Electro-Acupuncture, Traditional Chinese Herbology mixed with nutraceuticals, and Tui Na (Chinese structural alignment) are some of Dr. Corradino's special integration techniques. His passion, devotion, and belief in the integration of TCM and Western medical science contribute to his success.

Dr. Corradino has owned several clinics on hospital campuses and enjoys presenting the scientific research of the neuroscience of acupuncture to Western health care practitioners. He finds that they are extremely responsive. Dr. Corradino has developed Neuropuncture to better understand acupuncture's mechanisms, cross-reference these mechanisms to TCM theory, create an acupuncture system in which practitioners can illustrate reproducible, consistent, and successful acupuncture treatments, and provide a new understanding of this ancient art and medicine.

Abbreviations

Please make yourself familiar with the following abbreviations, which appear frequently throughout this book.

BL10	Urinary Bladder 10 acupuncture point
C1–5	Cervical vertebral bodies 1–5
CGRP	Calcitonin gene-related peptide
CNS	Central nervous system
CNV	Fifth cranial nerve
CNX	Tenth cranial nerve
DHA	Docosahexaenoic acid
EA	Electro-Acupuncture
EN	Electro-Neuropuncture
fMRI	Functional magnetic resonance imaging
GB21	Gall Bladder 21 acupoint
HT5–7	Regional area from acupuncture points Heart 5–7
HTJJ	Hua Tuo Jia Jie acupoints
L1–4	Lumbar vertebral bodies 1–4
LI4	Large Intestine 4 acupoint
MFTRP	Myofascial trigger point
MRI	Magnetic resonance imaging
NOS	Nitric oxide synthase
ONE	Orthopedic neurological evaluation
PAG	Periaqueductal gray
PANS	Primary afferent nociceptive system

PC6	Pericardium 6 acupoint
PNS	Peripheral nervous system
PUP	Pain Upon Palpation
REN12	Acupuncture point Ren 12
S1–4	Sacral spinal segments 1–4
SI19	Small Intestine 19 acupoint
SP10	Spleen 10 acupoint
ST36	Stomach 36 acupoint
SUD	Subjective Unit of Discomfort
T1–12	Thoracic spinal segments 1–12
TCM	Traditional Chinese Medicine

Chapter 1

Introduction to Neuropuncture's Theory and Development

Neuropuncture is a special system of acupuncture that combines neuroscience, other Western medical sciences, and current evidence-based acupuncture clinical research with the classical TCM acupuncture model. It is my belief that a deeper understanding of acupuncture's underlying mechanisms empowers the practitioner with knowledge in treatment. Once we understand these mechanisms, we can apply these findings in the area of diagnosis and treatment of pain cases, internal medicine cases, sports medicine cases, and orthopedics; and this is truly only the beginning. Understanding these concepts creates an extremely effective approach to modulating the nervous system. Finally, we can intentionally target specific receptors for the release of particular neuropeptides, reset dysfunctional visceral autonomic reflexes for improved organ function, and depolarize excited, overstimulated nerve roots for pain management. Neuropuncture works by predominantly targeting and stimulating specific neuro-tissue.

When we take a look back to 5000+ years ago when TCM was being developed, the physicians of that time did not have the understandings and advancements in the study of anatomy and physiology, cellular biology, molecular biology, molecular genetics, and especially neuroscience that we have benefited from in the past 75 years. When these new scientific models are applied to classical TCM acupuncture theory, the "Ah-ha" light bulb goes on, and a lot of the mystery and smoke clears away, revealing an absolutely amazing neuro-medical treatment modality. Neuropuncture is the outcome of the weaving of two very different but also very similar medical theoretical sciences: Traditional Chinese Acupuncture and Western neuroscience.

Acupoints, meridians, and neuroscience

Let's look at an example: LI4, He Gu, is a very popular acupuncture point in TCM with many functions and traditional indications ranging from any pathology in the face, teeth, throat, neck, stomach, and intestines, to specifics such as headaches, redness with swelling and pain in the eye, epistaxis, toothache, facial swelling, sore throat, contracture of the fingers, pain in the arm, trismus, facial paralysis, febrile diseases with anhidrosis, hidrosis, amenorrhea, delayed labor, abdominal pain, constipation, and dysentery (Cheng & Deng, 1999). Many texts refer to its benefits; for example, Maciocia (1989, p.376) notes that "it can be used in many painful conditions located anywhere in the body" and "it has a strong influence on the face and eyes…and is often used as a distal point when treating problems of the face, including the mouth, nose, and eyes." It is known variously as He Gu, Joining Valley, Uniting One's Mouth, Tiger's Mouth, and Holding Mouth (Bensky & O'Connor, 1991).

Acupuncture point LI4 is located in the dorsal interosseous muscle, between the first and second metacarpal bones; its deep position is in the transverse head of the adductor pollicis muscle

(Bensky & O'Connor, 1991). It has a radius of about the same size as a dime, nickel, or a quarter, depending on the patient. TCM uses a unique body measuring system to locate an indvidual's acupuncture points (from early times TCM observed differences in anatomy from patient to patient, just as this is confirmed today with autopsies, gross and molecular anatomy, and physiology). The TCM Large Intestine meridian travels up the radial side of the arm and into the face. When we apply all of these findings, we begin to understand the deeper mechanisms of LI4. What we find is that the afferent delta fibers of the superficial radial nerve travel under and through the classical TCM acupuncture point LI4/ He Gu, which is supplied by a dorsal branch of the radial nerve, and in its deep position by a palmar digital branch of the median nerve (Bensky & O'Connor, 1991). The radial branch, He Gu's main innervation, branches from and creates a large part of the brachial plexus of C5–T1 (Rohen, Yokochi & Lutjen-Drecoll, 2003). It also has A-delta fibers that terminate in the hypothalamus. When the hypothalamus is stimulated, beta-endorphins are released, which then stimulate the periaqueductal gray (PAG), creating a strong systemic pain-relieving effect (White, Cummings & Filshie, 2008). The fact that the brachial branch innervates C5–T1 tells us that all other nerve innervations will be affected at this spinal segmental location (see Figure 1.1).

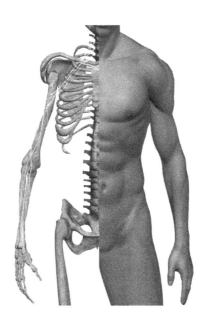

Figure 1.1 Radial nerve

Theoretical nerve physiology can be applied, and we notice that a range of conditions can be treated, ranging from cervical pain to facial pain, ear pathology, and eye pathology; and since that pathway influences the chest, cardiac and gastric conditions can also be treated. Therefore, it's no surprise when we look back and see that the single distal acupoint LI4/He Gu affects all these areas of the body and is used to treat so many different, same-side facial complaints, since the superficial radial nerve has an effect on the brachial plexus and together with the nerve branches, distal and terminal, exerts influence over the side of the head and face. Segmentation above the thoracic spinal column therefore, in accordance with neuroanatomical dorsal horn theory, will influence anything below that segment (White *et al.*, 2008).

In an effort to examine this further, we must not omit the fact that if we align a chart of the Yin meridians with a chart of the upper arm nerve pathways, they are almost identical (see Figure 1.2).

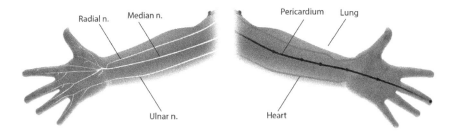

Figure 1.2 Upper extremity nerves and upper extremity acupuncture pathways

A re-analysis of all TCM acupuncture theory and TCM acupuncture classics such as *Huang Di Nei Jing* and *Ling Shu*, in conjunction with these neuroanatomy understandings, is necessary in order to catapult acupuncture into the future along with present-day medicine. It also means we can begin to understand acupuncture's unique and extremely powerful effects in the hope of maximizing these effects and expounding on them. Neuropuncture is the beginning of this process. It is important to understand that this does not take any credit away from classical TCM acupuncture, but only strengthens its value and appreciation due to its undeniable relationship with neuroscience and consistent clinical outcomes when applied. Examining the theory and art of TCM and tracing its patterns and cross-referencing them with modern-day neurophysiology and Western medical science as a whole is an integrative science that will truly help to enlighten this medical science and art. These classical TCM principles have achieved clinical success for thousands of years. Saying that we cannot understand all of the mechanisms does not dismiss its effectiveness in any way. We may not currently have a "complete" Western medical scientific explanation of all acupuncture's phenomena, but that only helps to encourage us to take a deeper look. Neuropuncture is the beginning of this journey.

Qi and afferent neurophysiology

The TCM classics state that the patient must feel the Qi sensation in order for the treatment to be effective. Some have interpreted this as meaning that the practitioner should feel the Qi grip the needle. Nearly every clinical trial and study completed today on acupuncture is performed with the protocol calling for the needle to be stimulated until De Qi ("Big Qi Sensation") has been obtained by the patient. There are two fascinating points of view to consider here and neuroanatomy underlies them both. The first is the De Qi sensations experienced by the patient, as explained in the *Nan Jing* (Unshuld, 1986) and *Ling Shu* (Wang & Wang, 2007). These classical sensations are: Ma (numbness), Chang (distension), Suan (an ache, muscular ache), and Chung (heaviness); also warmth, cold, the sensation of ants crawling on the skin, and slight pain (a prick). The second point of view of the De Qi sensation is that felt by the practitioner when needling and manually stimulating the needle. Qi has many translations, including vital breath, air, vapor, atmosphere, and energy (Jing-Nuan, 1993).

Many different styles of acupuncture require stimulating the needle with different needle techniques to stimulate the Qi in various ways, resulting in different effects (Cheng & Deng, 1999). The *Ling Shu* says: "Once the Qi has been reached, do not repeat" (Wang & Wang, 2007, p.332). This illustrates that the ancient masters of acupuncture were aware of the sensitive nature of the underlying neuroanatomy and that it was not to be harassed or insulted. Correlating the different De Qi sensations with different therapeutic actions (a warm De Qi sensation treats a cold condition) further shows that different Qi sensations were known to result in different physiological effects. This also illustrates the ancient practitioners' understanding that when Qi was felt, the stimulation was complete.

When an acupuncture needle is inserted into the desired acupoint, there are several different peripheral afferent fibers that can be found in the area of insertion. These are the true A-delta, A-beta, and A-gamma fibers in the skin, C-fibers, and II and III muscle fibers that create this neuro-network underneath the surface (Filshie & White, 1998). Patients report experiencing sensations such as pressure, tingling, radiating, spreading, heaviness, deep ache, and even traveling sensations. The free nerve endings of those small myelinated and unmyelinated fibers are organized into broad networks and produce sensations exactly like the ones that the masters in our classics report: light touch, pressure, vibration, numbness, deep pressure, heaviness in muscle, pinprick in skin, cold, soreness, aching, itch, and heat (Bensky & O'Connor, 1991).

These different sensations are directly associated with different neural tracts, with different terminal endings producing different outcomes. Also these tiny nerve fibers get wrapped around an acupuncture needle shaft during needle stimulation and give the practitioner the "grasped" feeling. At the local insertion site there can be up to 15 different neurochemicals, amino acids, cellular enzymes, and red and white blood cells, which produce a unique healing chemical soup (Filshie & White, 1998). So, to go back to LI4/ He Gu, we can stimulate that area differently, using different needle techniques, and produce several different sensations, stimulating several different nerve tracts and thus producing several different physiological responses to treat several different conditions. Also, as we mentioned, the superficial radial nerve travels up the arm and continues to merge with the brachial plexus and innervates C5–T1. This branch will affect all the nerve roots that merge and enter into the face, neck, and shoulder; some merge with cranial nerves that affect organs in the thoracic cavity, and all of these exit the cervical spine from C5–T1 (Marieb & Hoehn, 2009). So, indirectly, you can absolutely affect the facial nerves by stimulating the superficial radial nerve distal branch at LI4/He Gu, as well as affecting internal visceral structures while producing several different sensations (see Table 1.1).

Table 1.1 The neuroscience of De Qi

Classical De Qi sensation	Associated nerve fiber
Soreness	C-fiber
Numbness	A-gamma
Vibration	A-beta
Heaviness	A-delta, III muscle fiber
Achy	IV muscle fiber
Cold	A-delta
Hot	C-fiber, IV muscle fiber
Pinprick	A-delta

Neuropuncture has been in the "researching and organization" stage for the past 10+ years, and is still developing. I wholeheartedly believe that this material and its future work will enhance your understanding and practice of acupuncture, as well as aid in carrying you into the future of acupuncture in our Western and global medical science society.

Chapter 2
Review of Basic Neuroanatomy

In the neuroanatomy of the brain, a nucleus is a neural brain structure consisting of a relatively compact cluster of neurons. It is one of the two most common forms of nerve cell organization, the other being layered structures such as the cerebral cortex (or cerebellar cortex) and cingulate gyrus. The vertebrate brain contains hundreds of distinguishable nuclei, varying widely in shape and size. A nucleus may itself have a complex internal structure, with multiple types of neurons arranged in clumps (subnuclei) or layers, such as in the pituitary (Filshie & White, 1998).

The term "nucleus" is in some cases used rather loosely, simply to mean an identifiably distinct group of neurons, even if they are spread over an extended area. The reticular nucleus of the thalamus, for example, is a thin layer of inhibitory neurons that surrounds the thalamus (Marieb & Hoehn, 2009). It is these layers that have terminal ends that extend from the focal area of some acupuncture points (Filshie & White, 1998; White *et al.*, 2008).

Some of the major anatomical components of the brain are organized as clusters of interconnected nuclei. Notable among these are the thalamus and hypothalamus, each of which contains several dozen distinguishable substructures. These substructures explain the profound responsibilities and vast areas of influence these components have. The medulla and pons also contain numerous small nuclei with a wide variety of sensory, motor, and regulatory functions (e.g. breathing and cardiac). This is all contained in the central nervous system (CNS) and, respectively, the brain, but have neural tracts that feed information back to them from the peripheral (Marieb & Hoehn, 2009). Furthermore, the recent discoveries in neuroscience involving revolutionary concepts in neuroplasticity open new worlds for exploration and medicine.

Since acupuncture is performed on the peripheral of the CNS, let's examine the neuroanatomy relevant to that as well. The peripheral nervous system (PNS) has specialized structures that respond to changes in our environment. They are grouped as sensory receptors and include:

- exteroceptors, which sense stimuli arising outside the body

- interoceptors or visceroceptors, which respond to stimuli inside the body

- proprioceptors, which tell the brain where we are relative to other body parts' nociceptors, which respond to potentially damaging threats to tissue.

(Marieb & Hoehn, 2009)

These specialized groups of structures include nerve tracts, ganglia (clusters of neurons in the PNS), and specific receptors. It has been concluded from the imaging studies of acupuncture points that ganglia occur near or directly subdermal to many traditional acupuncture points (Marieb & Hoehn, 2009). It is at these Neuropuncture acupoints that ganglia are accessed, and the stimulation can be sent up tracts to specific regions of brain tissue, as well as to target specific spinal segments and plexuses.

Below is a short list of terms that need to be understood and conceptualized in order to grasp this system. I would encourage practitioners of acupuncture to undertake further studies in neuroscience, neurophysiology, neurophysics, or molecular biology and pharmacology as, in my opinion, to be a physician of acupuncture, you must first understand neuroscience. It is the micro and macro of acupuncture today! The following terms are explained and defined as they apply to this topic, but these are and by no means conclusive definitions.

- Central nervous system (CNS): The CNS comprises the brain and spinal cord. The brain is the central command center, and the spinal cord is a highway of neurotracts. The spinal cord is segmented by different levels of visceral and somatic neuro-innervations. Those innervations converge and travel up the spinal cord in tracts that terminate in specific regions of the brain, relaying information to the central command center.

- Brain: This is the central command center, the largest and most sophisticated pharmaceutical outfit in the world today. Even now it is not fully understood and is referred to generally as the "last frontier for medicine." Composed of 60 percent fatty acids and cholesterol, and 40 percent proteins, functional magnetic resonance imaging (fMRI) studies have revealed corrugations between very specific regions and areas of the brain with very specific functions and responsibilities in relation to acupuncture's mechanisms.

- Cerebral cortex: This is the folded, outermost, layer of tissue covering the brain. It is responsible for higher functioning in humans. Peripheral nerve stimulation (i.e. Electro-Acupuncture) sends nerve impulses along larger nerve tracts to reach the brainstem; they then fire up and stimulate regions of the cerebral cortex before terminating in other regions of the inner brain.

- Limbic area: This is a set of evolutionary primitive brain structures located on top of the brainstem and buried under the cortex. Limbic system structures are involved in many of our emotions and motivations, particularly those that are related to survival. Such feelings include fear, anger, and emotions related to sexual behavior. The limbic system is also involved in feelings of pleasure that are related to our survival, such as those experienced from eating and having sex. It also plays a major role in chronic pain.

- Hypothalamus: This portion of the brain contains a number of small nuclei with a variety of functions. One of the most important functions of the hypothalamus is to link the nervous system to the endocrine system via the pituitary gland (hypothalamo-pituitary-adrenal axis). The hypothalamus is located below the thalamus, just above the brainstem. In the terminology of neuroanatomy, it forms the ventral part of the diencephalon. All vertebrate brains contain a hypothalamus. In humans, it is roughly the size of an almond. The hypothalamus is responsible for the release of beta-endorphins. These endorphins in turn stimulate the PAG for systemic pain relief. The hypothalamus also controls body temperature, hunger, thirst, fatigue, sleep, and circadian cycles.

- Thalamus: This is a limbic system structure connecting areas of the cerebral cortex involved in sensory perception and movement with other parts of the brain and spinal cord that also have a role in sensation and movement. As a regulator of sensory information, the thalamus controls sleep and states of consciousness when we are awake, and also plays a role in pain management. The auricular acupuncture point exerts an influence and stimulates the thalamus for pain management.

- Cingulate gyrus: *Cingulum* is the Latin word for "belt." The name was probably chosen because this cortex, in great part, surrounds the corpus callosum. It receives input from the thalamus and the neocortex. It is an integral part of the limbic system and is involved with emotion formation and processing, learning, and memory. It is also important for executive function and respiratory control. It consists of the "folded layers of tissue" that along with the cerebral cortex help to make up 40 percent of the brain.

- Amygdala: The amygdala is an almond-shaped mass of nuclei located deep within the temporal lobe of the brain. It is a limbic system structure that is involved in many of our emotions and motivations, particularly those related to survival. The amygdala is involved in the processing of emotions such as fear, anger, and pleasure. It is also responsible for determining what memories are retained and where they are stored in the brain. It is thought that this determination is based on the size of an emotional response to an event. The amygdala is also a major area for sufferers of chronic pain and post-traumatic stress disorder.

- Pituitary: The pituitary gland is a small endocrine organ that controls a multitude of important functions in the body. It is divided into an anterior lobe, intermediate lobe, and posterior lobe, all of which are involved in hormone production. The posterior pituitary is composed of axons from the neurons of the hypothalamus. Blood vessel connections between the hypothalamus and pituitary allow hypothalamic hormones to control pituitary hormone secretion. The pituitary gland is termed the "master gland" because it directs other organs and endocrine glands, such as the adrenal glands, to suppress or induce hormone production.

- Periaqueductal gray (PAG): This is the part of the brainstem that is involved in pain suppression and is found in mammals. A large integral component for the endogenous descending pain system, it is stimulated by beta-endorphins, which are produced and secreted by the hypothalamus. There are certain Neuropuncture points with nerve endings that terminate in the hypothalamus and stimulate the secretion of beta-endorphins for pain management.

- Somatosensory regions: These areas of the cerebral cortex are responsible for the production of the sensory modalities such as touch, temperature, proprioception (body position), and nociceptive pain (the sensory nervous system's response to the experience of pain). We see direct relations with the classical scalp acupuncture motor and sensory lines.

- Primary afferent nociceptive system (PANS): These are specialized sensory nerve endings that include the A-delta and C-fibers. They are generally the first nerves to be involved in nociception. The system includes the network of A-delta fibers, retracing to the dorsal horn, up the spinothalamic tract, and terminating in the brain.

- Cervical plexus: C1–C4 is the nerve root plexus that exits the cervical spine at the levels of C1–C4, to become the lesser occipital nerve, greater occipital nerve, the transverse cervical nerve, and the supraclavicular nerve.

- Brachial plexus: C5–T1 is the nerve root plexus that exits the spinal column at the levels of C5–T1, which supply the arm.

- Lumbar plexus: L1–L4 is the nerve root plexus that exits the spinal column at the levels of L1–L4, which penetrate the lower limbs.

- Sacral plexus: L4–S4. The sciatic branch, L4–S3, is the largest nerve in the plexus and the entire body. S3 and S4 refer to the levels of S3 and S4 of the sacral fused vertebral bodies.

- Neurotransmitters: These are chemicals that are released by the axons and communicate and transmit information along a specific neuro-tract. There are many different types with vast responsibilities.

- Axon: Nerve extension that conducts impulses away from the soma (cell body).

- Dendrite: Nerve extension that conducts electrical impulses received from other neural cells.

- Resting membrane potential: Na++ (sodium ions) outside of the cell with K+ (potassium ions) on the inside of the cell. Negative inside versus positive on the outside (-70 mv).

- Membrane potential: Depolarization, a change on the resting membrane potential.

- All or none theory: Utilizing Electro-Acupuncture to bring about the action potential. This theory states that a nerve tract will change its membrane potential at a specific point of stimulus (-50 mv) and then anything after that point, or will not change at all.

- Descending pain system: The endogenous circuit that enables us to tolerate pain.

- Membrane threshold: -70 mv is the electrical charge required for a nerve cell membrane to hold before it changes its membrane potential, resulting in depolarization or repolarization of nerves.

- Myelin sheath: This is the lining around the nerve and consists of docosahexaenoic acid (DHA) molecules.

- **Opioid receptors:** G-protein-shaped neurons. Their stimulation releases endorphins.

- **Endorphins:** These are natural endogenous opioid polypeptide compounds—simply our body's natural pain killers.

- **Mu:** An opioid receptor with a high affinity for beta-endorphins.

- **Kappa:** An opioid receptor with a high affinity for dynorphins.

- **Delta:** An opioid receptor with a high affinity for enkephalins.

- **Beta-endorphin:** An endogenous poly-opioid peptide that regulates the perception of pain. It is produced and released by the hypothalamus.

- **Dynorphin:** An endogenous poly-opioid peptide that regulates the perception of pain. It has a high affinity to the kappa receptor. It is released from the hindbrain.

- **Enkephalin:** An endogenous poly-opioid peptide that regulates the perception of pain. It has a high affinity to the delta receptor and mu. It is released at the dorsal horn of the spinal cord.

- **Serotonin:** Biochemically derived from tryptophan, serotonin aids in down-regulating pain signaling from many locations of the body. Approximately 80 percent of the human body's total serotonin is located in the enterochromaffin cells in the gut, where it is used to regulate intestinal movements. This is another reason why we say "the stomach is our second mind." With regard to acupuncture and pain relief, we look at the specific release of serotonin at the dorsal horn.

- Afferent nerve fibers: Also referred to as sensory neurons, the afferent nerve fibers carry nerve impulses from receptors or sense organs toward the CNS.

- Efferent nerve fibers: Also referred to as motor neurons, the efferent nerve fibers carry nerve impulses away from the CNS to effectors such as muscles or glands.

- A-delta fibers: In acupuncture studies, this term refers to the broad section of A-gamma and A-beta fibers that create the neural network at the Neuropuncture acupoints.

- II and III muscle fibers: These are the fibers in the muscle that are responsible for some of the De Qi sensation in acupuncture stimulation.

- C-fibers: These are afferent nerve fibers found in the somatosensory system. They are unmyelinated and have a slow conduction velocity. They are mostly associated with "sharp" pain.

- Greater auricular nerve: Access to this nerve is via the Neuropuncture acupoint affecting C1–C5 of the cervical plexus.

- Radial nerve: The largest branch of the brachial plexus.

- Median nerve: A branch of the brachial plexus and the nerve injured in carpal tunnel syndrome.

- Ulnar nerve: A distal branch of the brachial plexus and the largest unprotected nerve in the body. It is felt when the "funny bone" is struck.

- Sciatic nerve: This innervates the spinal segment L4–S3. It bifurcates into the tibial, common, and deep peroneal nerves.

- Femoral nerve: This innervates the spinal segment L2–L4. It bifurcates into the saphenous and sural nerves.

- Peroneal nerve: This forms from the bifurcation of the sciatica nerve around the head of the fibular.

- Tibial nerve: This is the other bifurcation of the sciatica nerve.

- Femoral nerve: The largest branch of the lumbar plexus.

- Saphenous nerve: The largest branch of the femoral nerve.

- Sural nerve: A short branch of the saphenous nerve.

- Trigeminal nerve: This is the fifth cranial nerve (CNV). It is primarily a sensory nerve but it also has certain motor functions (biting, chewing, and swallowing).

- Vagus nerve: This is the tenth cranial nerve (CNX). The vagus nerve is responsible for such varied tasks as heart rate, gastrointestinal peristalsis, sweating, and quite a few muscle movements in the mouth, including speech and keeping the larynx open for breathing. It also has some afferent fibers that innervate the inner (canal) portion of the outer ear, via the auricular branch and part of the meninges. This explains why a person may cough when tickled on the ear (such as when trying to remove ear wax with a cotton swab).

- Calcitonin gene-related peptide (CGRP): This is the most potent peptide vasodilator and can function in the transmission of pain. Locally, for acupuncture purposes, it helps to vasodilate the surrounding capillaries to further release other powerful bio-chemicals.

- Nitric oxide synthase (NOS): An enzyme that produces nitric oxide from L-arginine. The neural type activates K+ channels, resulting in the hyperpolarization and relaxation of smooth muscles and nerves.

- **Myotomes:** A group of muscles whose supplied nerve is innervated at specific spinal segments and motor regions (see Table 2.2).

Table 2.2 Myotomes

Spinal exiting nerve	Muscle innervation
C1	None
C2	Longus colli, sternocleidomastoid, rectus capitis
C3	Trapezius, splenius capitis
C4	Trapezius, levator scapulae
C5	Supraspinatus, infraspinatus, deltoid, biceps
C6	Biceps, supinator, wrist extensors
C7	Triceps, wrist flexors
C8	Ulnar deviators, thumb extensors, thumb adductors
T1–T2	Minor innervations of intrinsic muscles of the hand, elbow, forearm, shoulder, scapulae, upper back, and neck
T3–T12	Innervations of the upper torso, as well as posterior and anterior aspects
L1	None
L2	Psoas, hip adductors
L3	Psoas, quadriceps, thigh atrophy
L4	Tibialis anterior, extensor hallucis
L5	Extensor hallucis, peroneals, gluteus medius, dorsiflexors, hamstrings and calf atrophy
S1	Calf and hamstring, wasting of gluteals, peroneals, plantar flexors
S2	Calf and hamstring, wasting of gluteals, plantar flexors
S3	None
S4	Bladder, rectum

- **Dermatomes:** Skin regions whose nerves are innervated at specific spinal segments and sensory regions (see Figure 2.3).

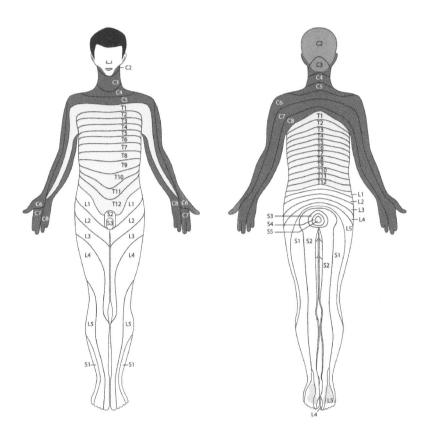

Figure 2.3 Dermatomes

- Viscerotomes: Organs and their spinal segment innervations (see Table 2.3).

Table 2.3 Viscerotomes

Spinal segment	Organ
T2–T4 (C3/C4)	Lung
T1–T5	Heart
T6–T10	Diaphragm
T6–T10	Stomach
T7–T10	Spleen
T7–T10	Pancreas
T7–T9	Liver and gall bladder
T9–T10	Small intestines
T11–L1 (to splenic flexure), L1–L2 (splenic flexure to rectum)	Large intestines
T10–L2	Kidneys
T11–L2	Bladder
T10–S3	Reproductive organs
S2–S4	Parasympathetic pathways of genital sex organs
T11–L2	Sympathetic pathways of genital sex organs
T10–T12	Ovaries
T11–L1	Fallopian tubes
T11–T12	Uterus
S2–S4	Vagina
L2–L1	Testicles
T12–L2	Prostate
L1–L2	Penis

Chapter 3
Neurobiology of Pain

Pain, whether it is in its acute or chronic stage, or emotional or physical, is one of the most common conditions treated with acupuncture. In fact, I believe that every acupuncturist and practitioner of Chinese medicine must treat pain on some level daily. Millions of people suffer every year, either from acute or chronic pain, and it is estimated that pain costs the USA $560–635 billion annually, half of which ($261–300 billion) is spent on health care costs (see www.painmed.org). Pain is one of the main reasons why patients are going to see their doctor—accounting for two out of every three reasons to visit.

There are many different techniques of acupuncture that have been developed over the years to treat pain using many different thought processes. We have advanced scalp acupuncture systems, auricular systems including battlefield acupuncture and P-Stim medical devices, Japanese style, sports acupuncture, orthopedic acupuncture, osteopuncture, and of course Neuropuncture.

I believe that in order to treat a problem you must first fully understand it. Pain is actually a specific area of our body's somatic sensory nervous system. The term "pain" is used to describe a wide range of unpleasant sensory and emotional experiences associated with actual or potential tissue damage. Remember that the terms "actual" and "potential" illustrate how pain is a subjective experience. Recent neuroscience research has illustrated that acute and chronic pain have neuroanatomical differences. Pain has been labeled a "neural signature" because it involves several areas of the brain, not just one specific region, depending on several variables. To best understand the neurobiology of pain I have broken it down into systems or neural pathways. These systems, or "orders," follow the transmission of pain from its origin.

Transmission of pain

Descartes first illustrated the neurobiology of pain in 1664 (see Figure 3.1). It was a rudimentary drawing of a simple pain pathway—the result of a flame burning the bottom of a man's foot. It depicts a line traced from the flame touching the man's foot, all the way up his leg into his "spine," then up to his head or "brain." The head/brain is where people believed the spirit got involved and gave the emotional component of pain. Interestingly enough, like our Chinese medicine predecessors utilizing the terms Jing Luo and Mai to describe pathways of transmission, Descartes wasn't that far off. The transmission of pain can be understood as following three main "orders" or systems of neurons, or simply three main neural-anatomical pathways. Let's investigate these pathways.

The first nerve order begins at the location of the actual or potential tissue injury. The human pain experience begins at this local site as a result of chemicals that are released transmitting information electrically to the CNS. Locally, there are tiny free nerve endings known as nociceptors. Nociceptors innervate everything from muscle, skin, and hair, to tendons, ligaments, bones, and viscera, and transmit information to the spinal cord.

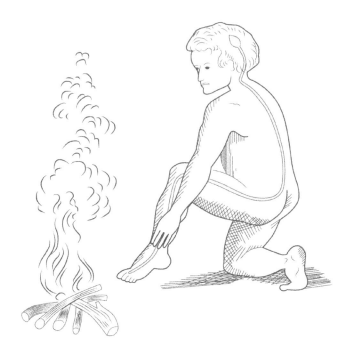

Figure 3.1 Descartes' pain pathways

Nociceptors include the A-delta, A-gamma, A-beta, and C-fibers. These tiny free nerve endings become stimulated via chemicals released locally as a result of tissue damage or an acupuncture needle being inserted into the skin. They transmit electrical signals of sharp pain, pressure, and variables in temperature. Thus, these fibers, which extend throughout our entire body, transmit everything—direct trauma, chemical damage, and temperature damage or changes—to our brain for interpretation and response. This system is known as PANS (see Chapter 2).

The local inflammatory mediators that are released include neuropeptides that have neural sources and non-neural sources. The non-neural sources include acetylcholine, adenosine triphosphate (ATP), glutamate, cytokines, some opioids, and serotonin. The neural sources include Substance P,

CGRP (see Chapter 2), neurokinin, choles kinase, somatostatin, glutamate, some opioids, and ATP. These neurochemical mediators all have an effect on specific receptors and they also affect the transducer channels such as the Na+, Ca++, and K+ channels. It is believed that these channels are directly affected by Electro-Acupuncture. Some of the chemicals are excitatory in nature and some are inhibitory. Together they are responsible for the transmission of pain.

This transmission continues directly to the spinal cord. The nociception fibers all enter the spinal cord at the substantia gelatinosa region of the lateral dorsal horn. This junction is where the transmission now enters the second order neuron of the pain neuroanatomical system. This junction is essential to pain transmission but also to acupuncture's powerful neurophysiological mechanisms. It is here that one of acupuncture's distal effects on the viscera and pain management can be clearly understood and explained (see Chapter 4). The different ways of stimulating the needle are what determine the message, which is transmitted as an electrical signal into a chemical one, then back into an electrical signal to the CNS.

It is at the lateral dorsal horn in the substantia gelatinosa that the "gate theory" applies. Since the C-fibers are unmyelinated and the A-gamma/beta fibers are myelinated and transmit faster, the signal transmitted by the A-gamma/beta fibers will block, or "gate," the area of transmission of the C-fibers. After converging, these tracts will penetrate specific regions of the brain but all together will affect the "pain signature" accordingly.

After crossing over to the opposite side, the spinal nerves all ascend to the brain. During its ascent to the brain the signal passes each spinal segment. There are several tracts that are involved. The stimulus, which then determines the tract, will determine the areas of the brain that will be stimulated or activated. Figure 3.2 illustrates the tract and the regions of the brain where the signal terminates its pathway. (Although this is a nice, neat, simple-looking diagram, it is in fact fairly complicated.)

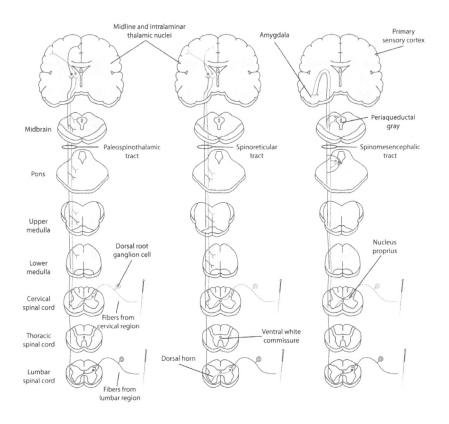

Figure 3.2 Ascending pathways along the spinal tracts

The transmission then continues into the brain and is now considered to be what neuroscientists call the "pain neural signature" or "pain matrix." Sometimes this anatomical activity is also referred to as the "pain neural substrate." It is a large, interconnected, complicated neural network that is still undergoing intense research. There are cortical and subcortical regions of the brain involved. The cortical areas include the somatosensory regions, anterior cingulate cortex, prefrontal cortex, and insula. The subcortical structures are the thalamus, amygdala, hippocampus, and basal ganglia. Collectively they form the pain matrix, which gives us the emotional and sensational experience and memory of pain.

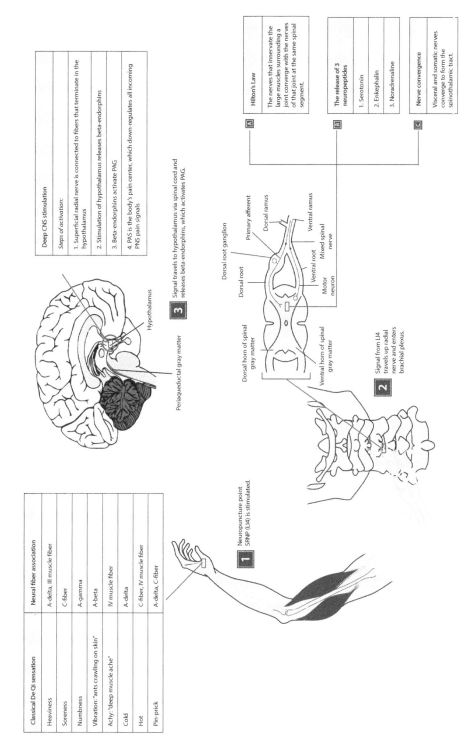

Figure 3.3 Neuropuncture clinical chart

Classification of pain

For classification purposes I break pain down simply into nociceptive pain or neuropathic pain, and pain with a peripheral or central location. Of course, for chronic and acute pain there are additional differences, with some neural anatomical variations, as we will discuss later in the chapter.

Nociceptive pain includes acute inflammation and myofascial pain while, separately, neuropathic pain includes neuropathies and radiculopathy. Neuropathic pain is separate because it involves different neurobiochemical factors as well as neuropathology.

- Nociceptive pain: In short, this includes PANS and the signaling of actual or potential tissue damage to the CNS— transmission from the peripheral local site to the spinal cord up to the brain. It also includes any inflammatory condition, which will activate the PANS but through specific inflammatory mediators. It also includes pro-inflammatory cytokines such as IL-1-alpha, IL-1-beta, IL-6 and TNF-alpha, chemokines, reactive oxygen species, vasoactive amines, lipids, ATP, acid, and other factors released by infiltrating leukocytes, vascular endothelial cells, or tissue resident mast cells. In addition, it includes muscle and joint pain.

- Neuropathic pain: This is a result of sensory deficits and abnormalities in the nervous system. It includes hyperalgesia and allodynia.

- Peripheral pain: This is due to an injury that originates outside the CNS, along the peripheral (e.g. arms, legs, ankles, hands, wrists, knees, etc.).

- Central pain: This is pain that becomes centralized in the CNS. It usually applies to spinal lesions, CNS tumors, and chronic pain.

I use additional combination classifications that are determined by the location of the source of the pain (i.e. a central or peripheral source). For example, peripheral neuropathic pain is pain in the peripheral of the body (pertaining to the extremities) that is also neuropathic. Pain over a period of time begins to change the brain, and just as the brain has the ability to mold and adapt to positive stimulation like meditation, in patients who suffer from chronic pain the structure of the brain changes but not in a good way. Changes occur that can be seen with fMRI and MRI images due to the consistent firing of neurons, which create, complicate, and increase the painful experience.

Next we will look at pain intensity and the time needed for diagnosis and treatment. It is important to remember that there are many well-recognized pain disorders that are not easy to classify and this can cause confusion in understanding their underlying etiology. Intensity helps us to understand the patient's experience of the pain signals. The time factor involves the practitioner understanding the area of the nervous system to address and focusing treatment in that direction.

Measuring the intensity of pain

I mainly use the Subjective Unit of Discomfort (SUD) in my clinic (see Figure 3.4). This method of clinical measurement requires the patient to grade their pain level at its highest and then at a constant. Level 10 represents pain so strong that they want to go to the ER and get an injection, and 1 represents pain that is barely noticeable.

- Mild: SUD 1–3

- Moderate: SUD 4–8

- Severe: SUD 9–10

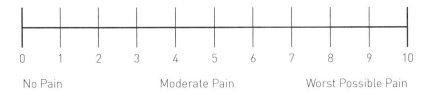

Figure 3.4 The Subjective Unit of Discomfort Scale

Another method is the Visual Analog Scale (VAS), which measures pain from no pain to extreme pain (see Figure 3.5). This can be better than the SUD scale because sometimes patients try to remember the last number they told you and want to adjust to that number. With a VAS, that scenario is eliminated and a more accurate reading is achieved. VAS is commonly used in research trials.

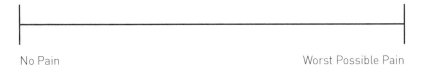

Figure 3.5 The Visual Analog Scale

Chronic pain

The last thing to discuss in this chapter is chronic pain complicated by chemical dependency. Recently there has been a focused movement by the US government to reduce the number of opioid prescriptions. Opioid addiction, opioid abuse, and opioid death have reached epidemic proportions. It can be a tricky process treating chronic pain and chemical dependency. You cannot just remove the addictive pain medication because the patient will be in severe pain and you cannot continue to increase the medication for risk of tolerance and then sudden death, or higher rates of addiction. It is a lot for the nervous system to handle. One of the most important things to remember, and to control, is the patient's anxiety level. During opioid cessation, it is common for patients to experience mild to severe levels at times, or a constant low level of feeling uneasy.

Auricular Electro-Acupuncture (EA) is very effective for opioid withdrawal. I use the National Acupuncture Detoxification Association (NADA) protocol in the dominant ear and then connect the Shenmen point in the NADA protocol to either the Tranquilizer or Lung point in the opposite ear and EA on 2 HZ millicurrent for 45 minutes. Remember to apply the Neuropuncture protocols at the end when necessary. So, for example, if the patient is experiencing hypertension, add the Neuropuncture hypertension protocol to the Neuropuncture anxiety protocol.

It is important to address the CNS when treating chronic pain. With chronic pain, the patient's brain molds and adapts to the stress of the pain signaling and needs to be "rewired" in many cases. This includes an integrated team approach, utilizing nutrition and mind–body training (e.g. meditation, psychology, and counseling), and Neuropuncture protocols that address brain health and the repair of specific neurons and neurogenic systems. Therefore it is common to treat patients every other day for several months to correct and "rewire" their nervous systems. This involves local treatment for the initial injury site, as well as focusing treatment on brain chemistry and CNS neural pathways.

Chapter 4

Neurophysiological Mechanisms of Acupuncture

To the age-old question "Where should the needle be placed, and how should it be stimulated for maximum benefit?" there is no one, single answer—it depends on what mechanism needs to be activated and what desired physiological outcome is determined. In this chapter we will look at five mechanisms: local, spinal segmental, endogenous opioid circuit, CNS, and neuromuscular.

1. Local mechanism

What is going on at the focal point of the acupuncture needle at the time of insertion and stimulation?

Why is it that when an acupuncture needle alone is inserted, incredible healing occurs locally? In Korea, a protocol has been introduced in which acupuncture needles are inserted all around the border and directly into second- and third-degree burns. This leads to incredible faster healing of the burn and much less scarring, if any, and results in little to no post-pathological neuropathy. I have utilized this theory style with tremendous success in the treatment of burns, post-op, stubborn, non-healing incisions, and skin infections. And why has simply inserting acupuncture needles directly into the plantar fascia resulted in the resolution of plantar fasciitis? How about needling around or directly into affected areas of slow-healing traumatic injuries?

At the site of the insertion, the special design of the needle (microscopically round, filiform, sterile, etc.) and the insertion technique produce a unique, healing, biochemical soup. The body's complex reaction to the simple insertion of an acupuncture needle is really quite remarkable. The instant an acupuncture needle is inserted, and then stimulated, an "axon reflex" occurs throughout the meshwork of surrounding nerves. This reflex results in the stimulation of specific fibers located in the terminal network of the primary nociceptive afferent A-delta fibers (including A-gamma and sometimes A-beta) and II and III muscle fibers. This in turn triggers the release of the CGRP (see Chapter 2), one of the body's most powerful vasodilators. This in turn dilates the surrounding local capillaries and leads to the release of other powerful neuropeptides. Locally, neuropeptides are released as a result of this local neuro-tissue stimulus. These chemicals have several specific therapeutic effects on the local tissues. It has been discovered that this local neurochemical accumulation consists of prostaglandins, red and white blood cells, glutamate, other excitatory amino acids, Substance P, and even serotonin from the local mast cells. This chemical soup begins to down-regulate the pain cascade, aids in reducing inflammation, starts the healing process of local and surrounding tissues, fights infections, and increases local circulation (Filshie & White, 1998; Marieb & Hoehn, 2009; White *et al.*, 2008).

There is an interesting technique I have learned and used called "osteopuncture." In this technique, you gently needle directly into accessible periosteum. This is a wonderful technique that directs that chemical soup to the bone level to treat such conditions as arthritis, stubborn fractures, ligament injuries, and shin splints. You do not needle deeply into the bone, just superficially into the periosteum or attaching ligament. The local chemical soup that is produced helps to heal bone injuries and ligament inflammatory injuries.

What is actually happening when a De Qi sensation has been obtained locally?

When a De Qi sensation has been achieved, we are certain that, based on the type of sensation the patient reports, we can determine which specific afferent sensory nerves have been stimulated. Those neuropeptides that are released locally (mentioned above) are what stimulate the afferent fibers and result in the De Qi sensation. Different needle stimulation techniques result in different sensations due to different neuropeptides being released as a result of the technique employed. The different techniques also have an effect on the amount of chemicals released (stronger techniques yield more). Hence different sensations lead to the stimulation of different afferent fibers and different outcomes. In other words, the local cutaneous afferent nerve fibers when stimulated elicit a specific sensation and reaction referred to as "axon reflex," which results with the initial stimulation of the "acupoint."

When we are training, our teachers constantly remind us, as do the TCM classics, of the importance of the De Qi sensation. For either the patient or we the practitioners feeling "the Qi gripping the needle," De Qi is important for the outcome of the treatment. We can now explain through neurochemistry what our patients are feeling, as described above, and it is an interesting fact that under electro-microscopic imaging a sterile, disposable, microscopically round acupuncture needle has been shown to grasp and wrap tiny nerve fibers (A-delta) around its shaft during rotation techniques, explaining why practitioners feel the "Qi grasping" the needle.

Here are some quotes from classical TCM texts that illustrate the connection between a De Qi sensation, needling, and the desired effective clinical outcomes:

> Needling is effective when one obtains De Qi. (*Ling Shu*, Chapter 3)

> Needling is effective when Qi arrives. (*Ling Shu*, Chapter 1)

> When the patient inhales, twist the needle to get De Qi. (*Su Wen*, Chapter 2)

Throughout my researching and reviewing of clinical trials on the efficacy of acupuncture in scientific environments, I have found that the more concrete findings, highest success rates, and consistent reproducible outcomes are achieved when the patient obtains a De Qi sensation. I have read in so many texts: "The needle was stimulated until a De Qi sensation was obtained." So, seeing that pattern and putting it into clinical practice and theory, we find a systematic approach to yield better outcomes.

The acupuncture needle can be inserted utilizing traditional hand insertion or guide-tube insertion. In either event, the needle after insertion should be stimulated until the patient feels a De Qi sensation. Remember, this should be a comfortable Qi sensation, not a sharp or stabbing/burning/painful sensation. A dull, achy, warm, heavy, distended, traveling, fullness sensation, or even a small muscle fasciculation, is fine. (Also, keep in mind that certain medications can amplify pain, such as with hyperalgesia.) As explained above, those classical sensations are the peripheral afferent nerve fibers firing and eventually hitting their mark: the brain and specific receptors. For a patient to feel those sensations, or any sensation for that matter, the afferent fibers of the A-delta, II and III muscle fibers, or C-fibers must have been stimulated (see Chapter 1 for the neuro-breakdown of De Qi sensations).

Table 4.1 Peripheral nociceptors and their transmitted sensations

Sensory fiber	Skin	Muscle	Sensation
Large myelinated	None	I	None
Large myelinated	A-beta	II	Light touch, pressure, vibration
Medium myelinated	A-gamma	II	Numbness
Small myelinated	A-delta	III	Deep pressure, heaviness in muscle, pinprick in skin, cold
Small myelinated	C	IV	Soreness, aching, itching, heat, calmness, second burning pain

Adapted from Filshie & White, 1998; White et al., 2008

One thing is clear: patients who report feeling a comfortable De Qi sensation yield better outcomes in scientific clinical trials and clinically. However, there is no need to overstimulate, or vigorously treat, to the extent that patients feel uncomfortable. There has been *no* scientific or clinical evidence of higher efficacy with excessive stimulation—actually the opposite has been recorded. The A-delta fibers and II and III muscle fibers are the target fibers. They are the fibers that transmit more pleasant sensations, because they have been known to have neural tracts that terminate in specific areas of the brain, and specific receptors, and they then release specific neurotransmitters when stimulated (White *et al.*, 2008).

This section has outlined the beneficial mechanisms behind local needling and provided a neural description of De Qi sensations. We can utilize this scientific evidence to needle locally with the sole purpose of creating a local, chemical, natural, healing soup!

Does every TCM acupuncture point have
this local healing potential?

For the local mechanism, the answer is quite often "yes." However, out of the 364 classical TCM acupuncture points, less than half have been evaluated and have a collection of neural tissue that when stimulated has a deeper, more profound effect on the nervous system and stimulates the CNS for a systemic, visceral therapeutic effect. The specific location of a TCM "acupuncture point" is difficult to determine. It is the neural tissue that we aim for, and although the classical location of TCM acupuncture points can give us a general area to examine, further understanding leads to accessing other areas of the body where this neurophysiological phenomenon occurs to access the inner workings of our elaborate nervous system.

2. Spinal segmental mechanism

For this mechanism, we examine the neuroanatomy of the spinal cord. We study where and how the peripheral nerves innervate the spinal segments and conclude with three important findings. First, it is important to recognize that all primary afferent nociceptive fibers (A-delta group, C-fibers, and II and III muscle fibers) enter the spinal column via the dorsal horn. Second, it is at this specific entrance that the somatic and visceral afferent nerve fibers converge and then cross over and travel up the same single tract (spinothalamic tracts, either paleo or neo). Third, these tracts terminate at various areas of the brain, yielding different neurological outcomes.

At the level of the dorsal horn, small intermediate cells are stimulated and the neuromodulator/endorphin, enkephalin, is released and blocks the transmission of pain in the substantia gelatinosa. Additional neurotransmitters are released at the dorsal horn of the spinal cord, namely serotonin and noradrenaline. These neurotransmitters have a general depression effect on the activity of the dorsal horn. This, in turn, immediately begins to reduce and modify the signaling of pain. So, we see segmentally at the specific level of neural innervation of the nociceptives that there is depression of the transmission of pain but also anything now under this level will feel the effects of the depression of the ascending pain system. This means that if you needle and stimulate an acupoint whose neuroanatomy enters the cervical spine, everything below that innervation will benefit from the depression of ascending pain signals. This effect takes some time to develop (10–20 minutes) but outlasts the duration of the stimulation and has been reported to last several days (Filshie & White, 1998; Marieb & Hoehn, 2009; White *et al.*, 2008).

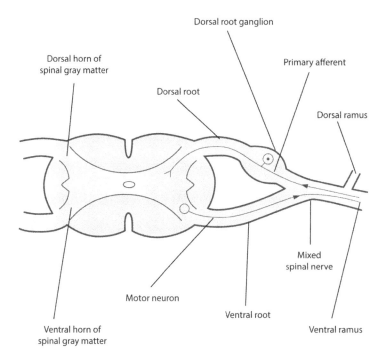

Figure 4.1 The dorsal horn

Visceral application

By depressing the dorsal horn activity, we affect both somatic and visceral afferent nerves because they converge at the dorsal horn into the *same* neurotract. What this does is inhibit any visceral dysfunctional autonomic reflexes of the leveled segment (Marieb & Hoehn, 2009). This results in the relaxation of the visceral smooth muscles. The relaxation of the visceral smooth muscle spasms will inherently release excessive, undesired stress on the targeted organ, increase healthy circulation, and aid in enhancing that organ's function.

Orthopedic application

Here we apply Hilton's law. The large muscles that surround and affect anatomical joints converge with those same nerves at the same segment of the spine. In this, one can modify the pain signaling from any joint. For example, the vastus medialis (SP10) is one of the large muscles that surround and affect the knee joint, as does the anterior tibialis (ST36). The nerves that innervate those muscles and the nerves that innervate the knee joint both converge at the second, third, and fourth lumbar vertebral segments. So, needling into these acupuncture points will directly affect the neurophysiology of the knee joint. How about the trapezius (GB21) and the splenius capitis muscles (BL10) and the cervical column and the treatment of cervical conditions? The trapezius muscles innervate the cervical spine at level C4–C5, as does the splenius capitis (Marieb & Hoehn, 2009; Rohen *et al.*, 2003).

It is important to remember that Neuropuncture acupoints have local effects as well as segmental ones. We can capitalize on *both* effects when needling and stimulating the points.

3. Endogenous opioid circuit (EOC) mechanism

Above we discussed the spinal segmental mechanism, which explained how the afferent nerve fibers, after being stimulated, travel to a specific level of the spinal segments and release enkephalins and other neurotransmitters, which depress the transmission of pain signaling. It is at these segments that the nerves that innervate muscles and the viscera also merge, affecting both directly. This impulse, or stimulation, does not end there. Acupuncture needling techniques also have an effect on our cerebral tissue. From the intermediate cells in the dorsal horn to the transmission cells, they then travel up the spinothalamic tract and have ends that terminate on the hypothalamus and other regions dependent on the acupoint. The hypothalamus is one of the largest manufacturers of beta-endorphins, which is another endogenous poly-opioid (natural pain killer). When the hypothalamus is stimulated, beta-endorphins are released that then travel immediately to the PAG (see Chapter 2). The PAG is simply the body's pain station. The beta-endorphins stimulate the PAG to depress all pain signaling that is being sent in from the peripheral.

We know that there are three main general groups of endogenous endorphins (the body's self-made pain killers). They are beta-endorphins, enkephalins, and dynorphins. Each of these groups has subsets but they are the three main endorphins that are mostly referred to in acupuncture research. They have affinities to specific receptors: mu, delta, and kappa, respectfully. We now also know that certain hertz with specific frequencies stimulate the specific release of targeted endorphins (Filshie & White, 1998; Marieb & Hoehn, 2009; Rohen *et al.*, 2003; White *et al.*, 2008). (Please see Table 4.2 and the protocols in Chapter 8.)

Table 4.2 Endogenous endorphin properties

Endorphin	Receptor	Frequency/amperage	Location
Beta-endorphins	Mu	2–4 Hz millicurrent	Midbrain/PAG/ pituitary
Enkephalins	Delta	2–4 Hz millicurrent	Dorsal horn of spinal cord
Dynorphins	Kappa	50–100 Hz millicurrent	Brainstem/spine
Orphanin	Mu	2/15 Hz millicurrent	Widespread

Source: Filshie & White, 1998

Serotonin is another neurotransmitter that acts as a powerful component in the pain control matrix. Serotonin also is released in the brainstem, which is involved in the descending pain inhibitory system. Not only does serotonin get released in the brainstem but it also stimulates the release of more serotonin in the dorsal horn, as well as noradrenalin. Both of these neurotransmitters strongly inhibit pain signaling in both directions. Now there is some evidence that certain pharmaceuticals can positively influence the effects of acupuncture. Tricyclic antidepressants increase the release of both serotonin and noradrenalin in the CNS. There is some evidence that these medications can amplify and reinforce the effects of acupuncture (Filshie & White, 1998; White *et al.*, 2008).

Neuroscience may help to explain, and legitimize, why acupuncture treatments have a cumulative effect, so that the patient receives better results the more they come. Opioid peptide metabolism illustrates that when there is a release of opioid peptides, there is also enhancement of gene expression, which leads to the manufacture of more opioid peptides to be stored at the terminal. So, when there is stimulation for a second time, the release is greater, resulting in a greater effect and better outcome.

The increased gene expression decays back to normal after about 3–5 days (White *et al.*, 2008).

4. CNS mechanism

We see several mechanisms for the effect of pain management with acupuncture via the PAG region of the brain. In addition, when the PAG is stimulated, the neural activity continues throughout the cerebral cortex, stimulating the thalamus, amygdala, and other centers of the brain. How does this affect its role on the immune system, drug dependency, endocrinology, nausea and vomiting, hypertension, and diabetes? All of these areas or conditions have been shown to respond favorably to acupuncture by the findings of fMRI and other imaging, illustrating how acupuncture neurophysiologically affects multiple regions of the brain, thereby correcting the pathology.

Immunology

Acupuncture in this area has only been recently studied, but the findings are positive. Possible mechanisms include generalized autonomic changes in the lymphoreticular system of the bone marrow and spleen. Also, the release of beta-endorphins into the bloodstream induces immune changes through the receptors on the leukocytes. There has also been evidence that acupuncture increases the natural killer cells, solubility of the IL-2 receptor, and changes in gamma interferon. Overall, what we discover does not provide a full explanation nor are the findings so far completely clear, but the area is promising.

Chemical dependency

There is an extensive amount of published literature in this area, particularly in the area of opioid dependency. The social effects are great and too political to discuss here. However, I have been told by professionals that, given the pharmaceutical opioid epidemic in the USA, we are now facing "opium wars" like the ones China experienced 200 years ago. The numbers of opioid addicts are staggering and reaching epidemic levels. So, with this in mind, let us look at how acupuncture can be applied to address this problem.

It has been shown that acupuncture is equally effective in many different areas of dependency or habituation. Auricular acupuncture has the most clinical and scientific research and has gained the most popularity. In the 1970s, China was utilizing auricular EA for opiate detoxing, utilizing bilateral Lung points in the concha, with EA for 30 minutes at 125 HZ millicurrent, for 2–3 consecutive days. The mechanism was at first thought to involve the stimulation of the vagus nerve that innervates the ear, resulting in a parasympathetic inhibition. However, there is yet another idea. Withdrawal symptoms are a result of an imbalanced adrenergic and cholinergic neurotransmitter system with an adrenergic predominance. So, EA actually stimulates the parasympathetic system back into balance. There is also evidence that EA also stimulates the enkephalins throughout the cerebral spinal fluid (CSF), resulting in a reduction in pain associated with a rapid detox. Chemical-dependent patients present significant alterations in extensive areas of the cortex (especially in the prefrontal and temporal cortex), subcortex (amygdala, hippocampus, and insular cortex), and basal regions (striatum). All of these areas have been researched and illustrate that EA stimulates these areas of the brain into homeostasis (Filshie & White, 1998; White *et al.*, 2008).

Endocrinology

As previously stated, it has been proven that acupuncture can stimulate the hypothalamus. From this stimulation, the anterior pituitary can be influenced and then the adrenals, which complete the hypothalamic-pituitary-adrenal axis. There is evidence that both adrenocorticotropic hormone (ACTH) and beta-endorphins are released with acupuncture. The hypothalamus is also the site for the production of the gonadotropin pulse regulator. This affects menstrual flow and timing, and it has been suggested that this is why acupuncture is so effective in women's health. Other studies suggest that the release of beta-endorphins modifies the CGRP, a strong vasodilator, which can aid in the reduction of hot flashes. 5-hydroxytryptophan (5-HTP) has also been proven to be released with acupuncture and this has a thermoregulatory effect.

Nausea and vomiting

This area has some of the most consistent positive outcomes in randomized clinical trials (RCTs) for nausea related to pregnancy, chemotherapy, and surgery. What has been consistent is the protocol ST36 (anterior tibialis), REN12, and PC6 (deep median nerve). This protocol seems to have an inhibition in emetic response and consistently produces positive outcomes.

Depression

D1 receptors of the prefrontal cortex have been shown to be stimulated with EA. There was a study concluded by the National Center for Complementary and Alternative Medicine (NCCAM) that illustrated a 90 percent success rate in the treatment of major depression (see protocols in Chapter 8).

Oxytocin

This has an interesting story. It was determined that infants nursing on their mothers' breasts sucked at a mixed rhythm. They would suck at one pace and then increase at one point, which resulted in milk being released. It was later discovered that this "peripheral" slow then faster stimulation on the mother's nipple stimulated the nervous system in a way that released the neuropeptide oxytocin from the brain. So, we apply a mixed frequency of 2–15 Hz, which mimics an infant breastfeeding and signals the brain to release oxytocin for many applications in obstetric and gynecological cases.

5. Neuromuscular mechanism

In the treatment of sport injuries and other orthopedic conditions, many times we are needling the MFTRP or motor points of large muscle groups, which stimulates the neural compartments of those muscles. What is actually happening when we needle these points? What we are stimulating is a specific neural loop, the PANS. These tracts have terminal endings throughout the limbic regions in the brain. When these acupoints are needled, they have a profound effect in relaxing and "resetting" the tight, wound-up muscle bundle. The local neurophysiological mechanism that produces the chemical soup also aids in the local healing of the muscle being needled. When these muscles are in spasm, they apply unnecessary pressure on the surrounding joints and tissues. When they are needled and "reset," they release static tension, and the undue pressure disappears. This also helps to stimulate the muscle's internal healing potential and fire neurons along its tract, leading to specific spinal segments and healing the entire "neural loop."

Chapter 5

Electro-Acupuncture

Science, Theories, Current Research,
and Their Clinical Applications

The subject of this chapter has been in practice since the 1930s and 1940s in China. We know traditional acupuncture has a history of approximately 3000–5000 years. It is just incredible to see how it has evolved with the advancements of science, into what we know now as "Electro-Acupuncture" (EA). Electro-Acupuncture was initially developed to replace manual stimulation and allow doctors to treat more patients. From that, EA has been modified with different frequencies, different wave forms, separate polarities, different currents, all having special effects on the nervous system. This research has led to today's design of evidenced-based protocols that target pathology directly. I use the term "Electro-Neuropuncture" for all of these applications brought together. That is, utilizing EA's scientific research and applying the neuroanatomy of acupuncture, and clinical experience, to create protocols with reproducible clinical outcomes. I would like to feel that the well-known Chinese medicine doctor Hua Tuo himself would be very proud.

In this chapter I am going to share with you the science of EA, how and when to best utilize it, and groundbreaking research that I am personally involved in that I feel will help change our profession and the world. I personally use EA on nearly every patient. I use it as an excellent way of focusing a healing electrical signal on the patient's nervous system in a way that communicates with that patient's nervous system. I see EA as physical therapy (PT) for the CNS, a treatment that balances, heals, and rehabilitates the damaged nervous tissue.

First the science: I have found that EA is either misunderstood or is simply not being utilized properly by acupuncture practitioners today. There are many common questions that I am repeatedly asked by veteran practitioners and students alike. Some that I always get asked are: What is the difference between millicurrent and microcurrent? Which frequency should I use for a specific condition? Which lead goes where—red and black? What are the contraindications? So, before I get into specifics, let's look at some basic physics to do with electricity. The main parameters that you should understand and differentiate between are the electric current, amperes, frequency, hertz, and voltage.

Current

An electric current is the *flow*, or *rate*, of the electric charge. This is the result of the effect of moving electrons. Voltage is the *energy* that the flow generates. In EA this movement is found inside the wires attached to the needles. This electric charge also generates an electromagnetic field locally, which has its own direct effect on humans. The international system of units measures current with amperes. So, when you see current and amperes, they are interchangeable. We acupuncturists tend to use the terms "microcurrent" or "microamps," and "millicurrent" or "milliamps." These are the two currents that I use in my clinical practice and that I will be discussing throughout the book.

Microcurrent is 1/1,000,000 of one ampere. Millicurrent is 1/1000 of one ampere. One ampere will illuminate an average household light bulb. These are very tiny charges. Nowadays all EA stimulator machines use AC voltage. AC stands for alternating current, as opposed to DC, direct current. DC means that the electrical flow is unidirectional—it flows only in one direction and can result in electrolysis. AC means that the electrical flow reverses periodically from one direction to the other. AC eliminates any risk of electrolysis and therefore reduces the risk of causing tissue damage.

Frequency

Frequency is the number of times the waveform completes itself in one second. Frequency is measured in hertz—1 Hz is one cycle per second. So, 15 Hz means that the waveform hits the needles 15 times per second. Increased hertz should not increase the sensation but can surprise patients. That is why I tell practitioners to begin with 2 Hz and then work up to 100 Hz in subsequent treatments. Always slowly and gradually increase the intensity dial until the patient can barely feel the stimulation. Then you can increase it until it is comfortably strong for maximum effect. Your patient should never feel pain or a burning or strong electrical sensation. Also, if you are using a mixed or burst stimulation—let's say 2–100 Hz—you want to increase the intensity while the 100 Hz is active. In this way you won't surprise your patient when the machine switches from 2 Hz to 100 Hz. One thing for sure is that the protocols I have listed in Chapter 8 are frequency specific.

Bi-phasic wave patterns

Bi-phasic wave patterns are important to understand as well. Bi-phasic wave patterns mean that the wave polarity switches from one direction to the other—positive to negative and the reverse. So, in reference to red and black leads, there is no scientific reason to place one color at any specific end; it is purely a matter of aesthetics *if your machine is bi-phasic.* They switch polarity, meaning the red or black leads truly do not indicate any specific charge. There are three machines on the market today that are FDA approved for EA, and they are the Pantheon, The Great Wall, and Ito. Pantheon is the only company that offers a bi-phasic wave form.

Table 5.1 Basic physical electrical definitions

Electrical qualities	Purpose	SI (International System of Units)
Electrical current	Charge of circuit	Amperes
Frequency	Cycles per second	Hertz
Voltage	Energy of circuit	Volts

As we discussed in Chapter 4, we now have confirmed specific frequencies that target specific neural receptors. What this means is that we have discovered that our nervous system responds to specific electrical frequencies. We can "communicate" with the CNS via electrical stimulation. We now know that at certain acupuncture points we can target specific areas of the brain and segments of the spinal cord to release specific neurochemicals and that this is all frequency specific. This is all made possible by simply understanding the neuroanatomy of the system, its response to electricity, and how and where to apply EA.

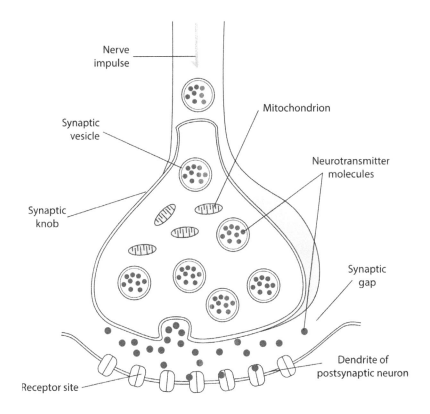

Nerve
impulse

Mitochondrion

Synaptic
vesicle

Neurotransmitter
molecules

Synaptic
knob

Synaptic
gap

Receptor site

Dendrite of
postsynaptic neuron

Figure 5.1 Neural synapse

Table 5.2 Endogenous opioid circuits (EOC)

Endorphin	Receptor	Frequency*	Location
NK cells	Immune	4 HZ	Widespread
Beta-endorphins	Mu	2–4 HZ	Mid-brain/PAG
Enkephalins	Delta	2–4/15 HZ	Dorsal horn
Dynorphins	Kappa	100 HZ	Brainstem/spine
Orphanin	Mu	2/15 HZ	Widespread CNS
5-HTP	5-HTPr	20–50 HZ	Hypothalamus
Oxytocin	OXTR	2–15/30 HZ	CNS
Dopamine	D1	2, 15–30 HZ	Prefrontal
NOS	Epithelium	2, 15–30 HZ	Widespread

* All frequencies are millicurrent.

Clinical EA settings and utilizing mixed frequencies, especially in the treatment of pain

So, for many, there is always a question of when to use microcurrent vs. millicurrent, and which frequency to apply and how intense should the stimulation be. I want to use this section to review a clinical application that I have found to be effective when applying EA stimulation. I utilize this theory when mainly treating pain cases that require mixed frequencies from low to high. The theory that research has produced in EA is that microcurrent has the ability to penetrate cellular walls and increase cellular respiration by increasing ATP production. This helps to heal tissues, especially soft tissue. So, I always begin using 25 HZ microcurrent to initiate and support the healing process of the local tissues and reduce inflammation.

I will continue this up to 2–4 treatments, depending on the patient's response. If the patient is responding well then why "fix something that is not broken," and I will continue until the condition is resolved. If it is time to change to millicurrent, then I will increase the stimulation to 2 Hz millicurrent at the following session. I will continue this for several treatments. I will then change the setting to 2–15 Hz for a mixed, or burst, stimulation effect, for a few treatments, then go to 2–30 Hz, and finally end up at 2–100 Hz (see Table 5.3).

Table 5.3 Sample Electro-Acupuncture treatment protocol

Treatment	Frequency	Current	Time interval
1–2	25 Hz	Micro	25–45 min
2–3	2 Hz	Milli	25 min
3–6	2–15/2–100 Hz	Milli	25 min

Theories of Electro-Acupuncture's effects

In this section I would like to share with you groundbreaking research and theories that help to explain EA's powerful effects. These theories are scientifically fascinating and are currently leading research in the area of EA and spinal nerve regeneration, oncology-electrochemotherapy, and EA-induced stem cell proliferation. These theories are in the process of mouse model clinical trials in Southern California by the International Association for Research of Electro-Acupuncture (IAREA). The team consists of a group of physicians,[1] Eastern and Western, who have come together in their own time to help gather and conduct EA research and establish a platform for international relationships between EA researchers.

I personally have seen much more successful research being done in EA than in straight manual acupuncture, and I therefore focus my own investigations on EA. The fact that EA protocols can be further quantified by time, specifically calibrate the

---

[1]   Members of the IAREA team are: James Dunn, MD, PhD; Duong Ha, L.AC.; John Hubacher, MA; Michael Corradino, DAOM, L.AC.; and Laura Kelly, DAOM, L.AC.

amount of stimulation, and are reproducible makes things easier for research and clinical applications. EA has also been shown to maximize acupuncture's effects and produce the most benefit, so this is another reason why I have chosen to research this specific area of acupuncture and share what I have found with you. There are five main theories that IAREA is currently discussing and researching. I believe that using these theories, and the neurophysiological mechanism described earlier, we can explain all of EA's effects and in some cases we can combine theories to support the conclusive data. Below I will list each theory, explain it in simple terms, and give an example of how it can be used, or where it may be applied. All of these theories are evidence-based and scientifically rooted.

1. Stem cell theory

With an MD and PhD in quantum mechanics, both from Harvard medical school, Dr. James Dunn is the leader of stem cell theory. Dr. Dunn is investigating the proliferation of stem cells after an EA treatment. He hypothesizes that the electrical stimulation communicates on a quantum level to release more stem cells for healing. Its application is of particular interest where tissue regeneration is needed. Dr. Dunn is a pediatric surgeon and is interested in utilizing this technique to help treat children who have been born with a portion of their small intestine missing. We hope to discover an exact protocol to aid in communicating with a child's stem cells to heal and regenerate the bowel without surgery, or perhaps assist in the healing post-surgery.

One of our goals is to determine the "amplitude window," or "frequency window," of the stem cells' cellular wall. This information will give us a direct electrical protocol that will specifically target stem cells, resulting in a proliferation of these stem cells for amazing clinical applications.

2. Antioxidant theory

Dr. Duong Ha first brought this theory to my attention. A free radical is a negatively charged particle that severely damages human tissue. It has a negative charge because it lacks an electron but it has the potential to gain an electron and become stable, which reduces its harmful effect on live tissue. An antioxidant is a particle that lends or donates an electron to the free radical and therefore stabilizes it. In our research we are trying to measure the human voltage prior to an EA session and then again afterwards to see if there is a measurable difference. Dr. Duong Ha hypothesizes that we are adding electrons to the human body and that the additional electrons act systemically as antioxidants. The question is, which acupuncture points and which frequency and hertz are best to potentiate the delivery of these free electrons to act as antioxidants?

3. Modified "gate theory" (gating the notch) mechanism

Dr. Laura Kelly, who works with spinal cord injury and paralysis, presented this theory to me. The theory is that when there is a spinal cord injury the human body will respond with a "notch signaling mechanism" that blocks the body's innate healing abilities from healing the damaged nerves. From her experience of reversing paralysis, Dr. Kelly believes that EA stimulation has a "gate theory" application on this notch signaling pathway. Where the EA blocks the notch signaling mechanism, the spinal nerves heal (i.e. the electro-stimulation inhibits the notch signaling pathway and promotes neural stem cell proliferation which heals the spinal cord lesion). See the Kelly Protocol at the end of this chapter. IAREA will be conducting mouse model trials to evaluate and measure the effect of EA on stem cells.

4. Electromagnetic field theory

This is a simple application of electromagnetism to EA that I stumbled upon myself. Wherever electricity is traveling along a metal wire, an electromagnetic field is produced. So, when we attach leads to our acupuncture needles, we are generating a local electromagnetic field around the needle. This I particularly apply to scalp acupuncture. I love utilizing EA on scalp points! In the Neuropuncture protocols where I use scalp points, it is this mechanism that I am applying. This is similar to transcranial electromagnetic stimulation. I have even seen research where EA of the scalp is termed "DCEA—deep cranial electro acupuncture" (Bun, 2014). This type of scalp EA has the same effects as transcranial electromagnetic stimulation does on the brain. It helps to increase blood circulation locally, increases neural activity locally, and helps to heal and regulate cerebral electrical activity. So, if you want, or need, to target the prefrontal cortex, then with an acupuncture point prescription like GB14 to ST8, or ST8 to Taiyang and applying EA, you will. I think this really opens up scalp acupuncture's application, especially when reviewing the scalp lines and their associated cerebral regions. It is no coincidence that the scalp acupuncture lines are directly over that region of the brain that they treat.

5. Frequency-specific concept—Hilton's law/stimulating the CNS/PNS via millicurrent and microcurrent

By now you will be aware of EA affecting specific receptors with specific frequencies. This research has been going on since the 1950s. Today we have a very nice understanding of how, when, and where to apply different frequencies to affect specific neural tissue. Research has confirmed the outcomes of the effects of specific frequencies, with specific amps, on specific tissue. For example, is has been confirmed that a 2 HZ millicurrent has the targeted effect on the mu opioid receptor at certain neural anatomical acupuncture points. A 100 HZ millicurrent has the effect of targeting the kappa receptor located in the dorsal horn of the spinal column and affects the enkephalin endogenous endorphin system. Notice they are both millicurrents. In addition, a 2 Hz millicurrent has been shown to help with IgG (immunoglobulin class G) factors and NOS blood levels, 2–15 Hz has been shown to increase fallopian tube blood circulation, and 100 Hz has a neuroprotective effect on the brain. (For protocols, please see Chapter 8.)

When reviewing research with microcurrent, we come across an interesting finding. For starters, the results are always intracellular, affecting cellular organelles. At 25 Hz microcurrent, it has been confirmed that the waveform penetrates the cellular walls and stimulates the mitochondria and stimulates ATP production. This is the mechanism that I have found which explains the findings in many clinical studies, and which is currently being researched. It illustrates the effect of the size of the waveform on the cellular wall and its penetration ability. It is clear that if this waveform penetrates the cellular wall and stimulates the mitochondria, then this same waveform may also have the effect of signaling the generation of the stem cells.

We can also target specific spinal segments with EA by utilizing the dermatome and myotome charts and needling acupuncture points within those areas. EA will also help us to utilize Hilton's law. By needling major acupuncture points, or motor points of the large muscles that surround a joint of focus and applying EA, we can then affect that joint directly via Hilton's law.

Oncology cellular wall permeability research: "Electrochemotherapy"

Cancer has been described as a dysfunction of electromagnetism on a cellular level. It can be seen as an invasion into the surrounding intracellular organelles as it affects multicellular systems. The loss of adhesiveness plays a major role in cancer's metastatic properties. The electrostatic interaction with positively charged atoms at the outer surface could change protein conformation (Pokorny, 2008). It is at this level of focus that EA has an effect. Electrochemotherapy utilizes a cytotoxic chemical in the body and then applies electricity, which changes the cellular membrane and allows the chemotoxic agent into the cells. What IAREA is looking for is the best frequency and hertz to aid in the penetration of cancer cellular walls—this is termed the "frequency window," or "amplitude window," and will give us the most effective wave form, frequency, current, and time interval.

This is a very important area for me. I am currently involved in the treatment of children who have been diagnosed with diffuse intrinsic pontine plioma (DIPG). DIPG is a devastating, aggressive brain tumor found in children. It arises in the pons, a region of the brainstem involved in critical body functions. Though brainstem tumors are extremely rare among adults, they comprise approximately 10–15 percent of all pediatric brain tumors. What seems to be the issue is that there is a 100 percent mortality rate for children diagnosed with DIPG. They cannot find a way for the chemotherapy to pass the blood brain barrier and target the cancer. I am therefore working on developing a protocol that will possibly assist in opening channels with EA so that the chemotherapy can permeate the brain and have its desired effect. There is also an EA protocol that I use that increases the "natural killer" cells of our immune system, as well as the IgG factors. I am working on combining techniques and protocols for the best reproducible outcomes.

Brenda Golianu, MD, and Elizabeth Sebestyen, MD, have illustrated that placing acupuncture needles in the "meridians" that travel through the cancerous tumor 1–2 cm proximal to the tumor border, and needling major acupuncture points distal along the same "meridians" and applying 2 HZ millicurrent for 30 minutes, affects the cellular walls of the tumor and definitely potentiates the chemotherapeutics' effect on shrinking the tumor (Golianu & Sebestyen, 2007).

Contraindications of Electro-Acupuncture

Always listen to your patients. Remember that we are looking for a comfortable, strong sensation (nothing burning or painful). This is what I call the "EA De Qi." Be sure never to overstimulate and never create any discomfort during treatment. As you have seen and will see with the Neuropuncture protocols, I always cross the spine, cross the head, and even needle into the spinal dura space. You must just be careful, use your common sense, and remember the following:

- *Do not EA through* an area of the body where there is any electrical device (e.g. pacemakers, medical pumps, spinal stimulators).

- *Caution* with EA around metal hardware.

- *Always* use clean needle technique, and use betadine and/or exam gloves when necessary.

- *Caution* with millicurrent on the face. Microcurrent is safer and effective.

- *Caution* with epilepsy. Never overstimulate the head and do not cross the brain with any scalp protocols.

- *Caution* with pregnancy.

- *Do not use* on any patients who have had electrical trauma (e.g. torture victims, those who have suffered electrical or lightning accidents).

The Kelly Protocol
Dr. Laura Kelly, DAOM, L.AC.

This protocol consists of five steps, to be applied three times a week for up to six months. It is aimed at healing spinal cord lesions including overriding the notch reaction. The theory is that the 25 Hz millicurrent blocks the internal natural noxious signal and allows the body's natural healing mechanisms to take effect (basically bypassing the signal, or "gating" the noxious notch signal). We have seen this effect clinically in the area of spinal cord injury and paralysis, chronic pain, and with interrupting dysfunctional visceral autonomic reflexes through the spinal segmental Neuropuncture mechanism. The gauge of needle can vary; I use 25 gauge 6 cun needles. Needle placement is illustrated in Figure 5.2.

1. Electrode placement in this case 1 x 6 cun needle into the epidural space at L3, preferably down into the epidural spaces of L4 and L5.

2. Electrode placement in this case 1 x 1 cun needle into all sacral foramen.

3. Electrode placement in this case 4 x 6 cun needles into the epidural space at T12, T8, T4, and T1.

4. Electrode placement in this case 1 cun needles into splenius capitis, splenius cervicis, and longissimus thoracis at C3, C6, T3, T6, T9, T12, L3, and L5, both sides.

5. Simultaneous manipulation of affected limb, either through manual therapy or preferably through assisted movement such as the adapted exercise bicycle as created for the protocol.

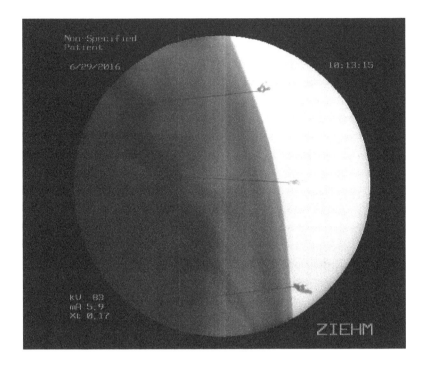

*Figure 5.2 Fluoroscopy image of the Kelly Protocol for
needle placement*

Chapter 6

Neuropuncture Acupoints

It is important to embrace a mindset of "neuroscience" when locating and needling Neuropuncture acupoints. Some of these points are near or directly under traditional TCM acupuncture points; however, you must learn to adapt a mindset of neurophysiology or you will completely miss the concept and have difficulty achieving optimal results. Remember, 2500+ years ago there was no advanced imaging science like we have today and no understandings of molecular sciences. People did not even perform any autopsies due to cultural respect for their ancestors, and as a result, they had less understanding of neurology and the neurosciences. What is truly amazing is that when we compare the findings of Neuropuncture and neurophysiology to traditional acupuncture systems, we can appreciate our predecessors' developed and keen powers of observation. Through my research into different needle techniques and differentiating De Qi sensations, I have realized that they were observing different neural receptors and afferent neural tracts. The location of the traditional meridians and the pathways of nerves all illustrate the tedious examination process our predecessors employed to develop the type of acupuncture we know today.

When performing acupuncture, I firmly believe that we must embrace the sciences and apply more neuroscience, because that is exactly what we are influencing. We are masters of manipulating and modulating the nervous system. Our nervous system communicates with every cell in our body and controls every bodily function. Using the ancient art of acupuncture, we insert needles into acupoints distal from the brain and then attach clips and send specific electrical messages through these acupoints to communicate directly with the brain, resulting in profound physiological balancing.

When compiling the actions and indications for the following Neuropuncture acupoints, I chose to list the neurophysiological understandings and conditions I often treat clinically. In this respect, I follow the laws of neuroscience; however, it is difficult to list the applications for balancing all the individual neurological pathologies that can potentiate, from pain to visceral dysfunction, so I compare "neurological deficits," from depolarizing said nerve tracts, to accessing the terminal receptors, and all the pathologies that can exist from within these parameters. That is the beauty of Neuropuncture: the ability to treat Western medical diagnoses by interpreting them with neuroscience pathologies and treating them accordingly. That is exactly what Neuropuncture is. That is why I associated the Neuropuncture acupoints with conditions I have utilized successfully in my clinic.

The acupoints listed on the following pages have been presented with the name of the Neuropuncture acupoint, then the nearest associated TCM acupoint, major nerve innervation, spinal segment (where the nerve connects to the spinal column when applicable), and conditions that have been successfully treated. Conditions treated can be applied to many other pathologies than those that are listed.

There is a saying in martial arts: "Learn the form, to grasp the technique. Grasp the technique and forget the form." Once you understand the application and the underlying neuroscience, then the applications are vast. Apply the following neuroscience information to your present tcm acupuncture protocols and try to grasp a deeper understanding of your treatment and gain further insight into your treatment mechanisms.

This table shows you where to find the Neuropuncture acupoints in the section that follows.

Neuropuncture acupoint	Location
Greater auricular	page 82
Infraorbital	page 84
Supraorbital	page 86
Tri-facial	page 88
Greater occipital	page 90
Lesser occipital	page 92
Spinal accessory	page 94
Lateral antebrachial	page 96
Deep radial	page 98
Superficial radial	page 100
Deep median	page 102
Ulnar	page 104
Carpal tunnel release	page 106
Saphenous	page 108
Tibial	page 110
Common peroneal	page 112
Sural	page 114
Medial popliteal	page 116
Deep peroneal	page 118
Posterior superior iliac spine (PSIS)	page 120
Paraspinal	page 122

The Primary
Neuropuncture Acupoints
(from the head to the extremities)

Greater auricular
Neuropuncture acupoint

TCM CLASSICAL ACUPUNCTURE POINT VICINITY	Approximately 0.5 in inferior to San Jiao 17.
BRANCH NERVE	Greater auricular nerve. Located at the posterior border of the ascending mandible.
SPINAL SEGMENT INNERVATION	C1, C2, C3, C4.
AREAS OF INFLUENCE	Ears, eyes, lateral posterior neck, throat, temperomandibular joint disorders, eye, facial nerve, auricular branch of vagus.
RELATIVE CONDITIONS	Said nerve deficits: *any* cervical conditions, tinnitus, ear pathology, migraine, temperomandibular joint disorders, trigeminal neuralgia, upper extremity paresthesia, headaches.

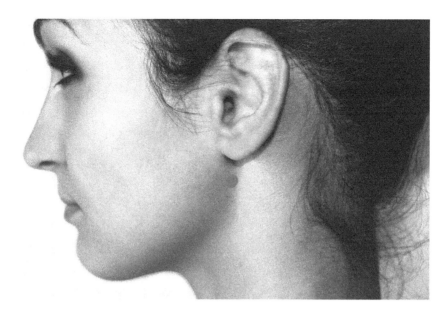

Figure 6.1 Greater auricular Neuropuncture acupoint

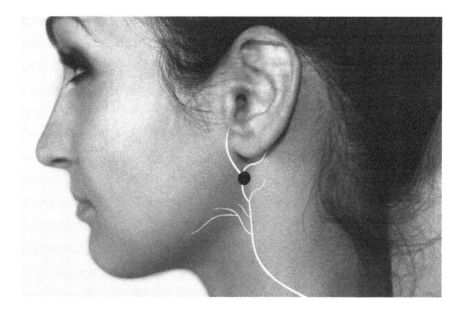

Figure 6.2 Greater auricular nerves

Infraorbital
Neuropuncture acupoint

TCM CLASSICAL ACUPUNCTURE POINT VICINITY	sT2–Qixue.
BRANCH NERVES	Infraorbital nerve and small branch of the facial nerve. Located in the infraorbital foramen.
SPINAL SEGMENT INNERVATION	Distal branch of the maxillary nerve/facial nerve and the third branch of the trigeminal nerve.
AREAS OF INFLUENCE	Infraorbital ridge pain, lower lid palsy, maxilla, maxillary nerve, trigeminal nerve, facial pain anywhere in the area from the lower eye lid, along the nose, to the upper lip of the mouth.
RELATIVE CONDITIONS	Bell's palsy, facial paralysis, eye pain, headaches, migraines, mouth pain, sinus pain and conditions, temperomandibular joint disorders, trigeminal neuralgia, stroke.

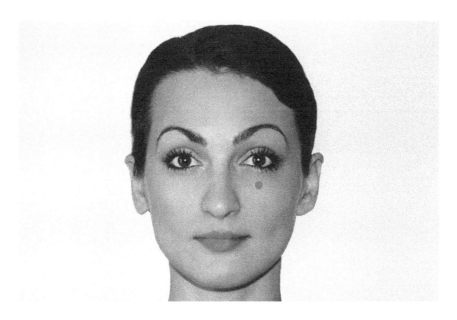

Figure 6.3 Infraorbital Neuropuncture acupoint

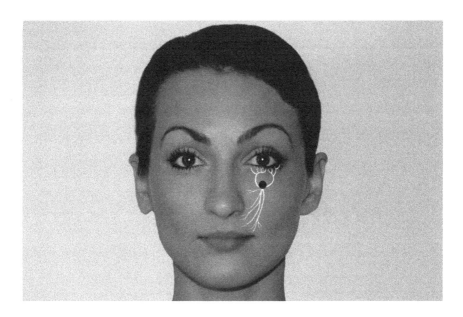

Figure 6.4 Infraorbital nerves

Supraorbital
Neuropuncture acupoint

TCM CLASSICAL ACUPUNCTURE POINT VICINITY	Slightly inferior to the extra TCM acupuncture acupoint named Yu Yao. In the supraorbital foramen, palpate for the supraorbital nerve.
BRANCH NERVE	Supraorbital nerve.
SPINAL SEGMENT INNERVATION	First division of the trigeminal nerve, the ophthalmic nerve, then further to split into the frontal nerve and then into the supraorbital nerve.
AREAS OF INFLUENCE	Supraorbital ridge, eye, head, face.
RELATIVE CONDITIONS	Bell's palsy, superior eye lid droop, headache, migraine, visual disturbances, pain anywhere from the upper eye lid to the forehead and scalp, reaching as far back as the lambdoidal suture.

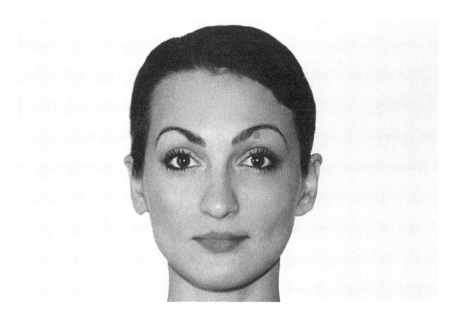

Figure 6.5 Suprarorbital Neuropuncture acupoint

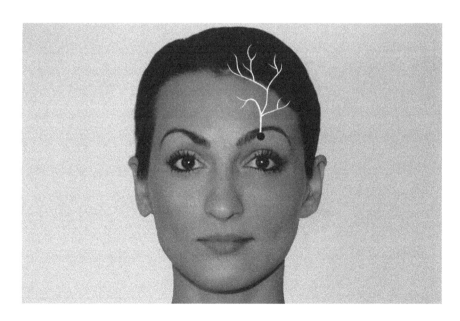

Figure 6.6 Supraorbital nerves

Tri-facial
Neuropuncture acupoint

TCM CLASSICAL ACUPUNCTURE POINT VICINITY	SI19/GB2/SJ21 region.
BRANCH NERVES	Trigeminal nerve, facial nerve.
AREA OF INFLUENCE	Entire side of face.
RELATIVE CONDITIONS	Trigeminal neuralgia, temperomandibular joint disorders, headaches, migraines, tinnitus, ear pain, facial paralysis, stroke, eye pathology.

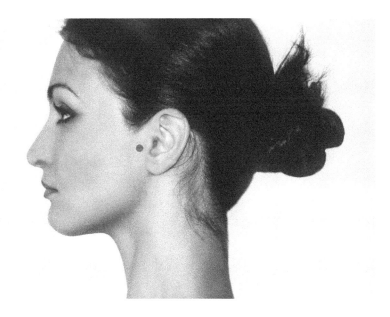

Figure 6.7 Tri-facial Neuropuncture acupoint

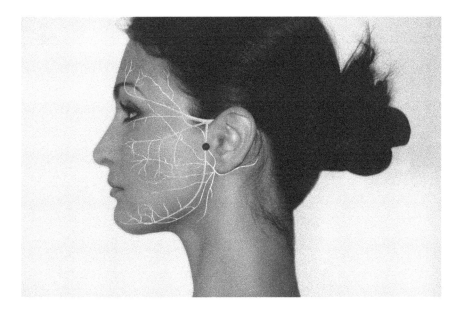

Figure 6.8 Tri-facial nerves

Greater occipital
Neuropuncture acupoint

TCM CLASSICAL ACUPUNCTURE POINT VICINITY	BL10. 0.5–1 in lateral to external occipital protuberance. Careful palpation will reveal its location.
SPINAL SEGMENT INNERVATION	C2.
AREAS OF INFLUENCE	Occipital region, posterior cervical muscles, trapezium, shoulder.
RELATIVE CONDITIONS	Migraines, headaches, trapeze conditions, cervical conditions, shoulder conditions, depression.

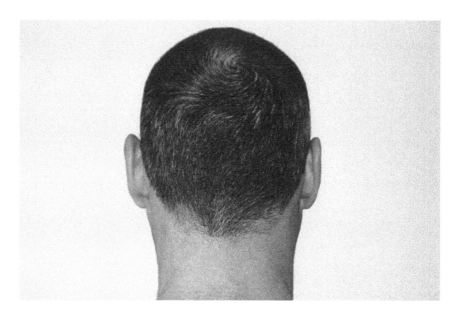

Figure 6.9 Greater occipital Neuropuncture acupoint

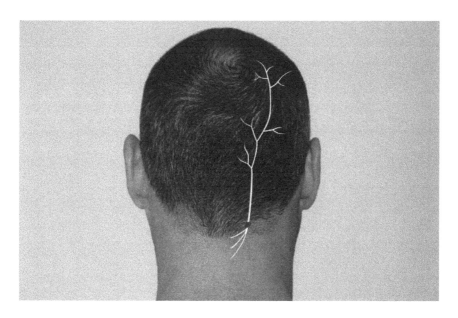

Figure 6.10 Greater occipital nerves

Lesser occipital
Neuropuncture acupoint

TCM CLASSICAL ACUPUNCTURE POINT VICINITY	GB20–Feng Chi.
SPINAL SEGMENT INNERVATION	C2.
AREA OF INFLUENCE	Communicates with greater auricular nerves.
RELATIVE CONDITIONS	Migraines, headaches, trapeze conditions, cervical conditions, shoulder conditions, depression.

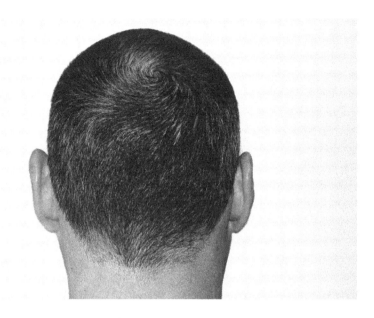

Figure 6.11 Lesser occipital Neuropuncture acupoint

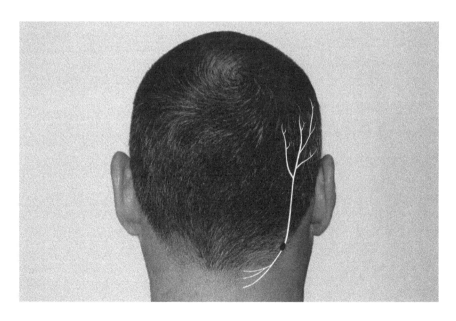

Figure 6.12 Lesser occipital nerves

Spinal accessory
Neuropuncture acupoint

TCM CLASSICAL ACUPUNCTURE POINT VICINITY	Posterior and inferior to GB21.
SPINAL SEGMENT INNERVATION	Cranial nerve XI. The spinal accessory nerve provides motor innervation from the CNS to two muscles of the neck: the sternocleidomastoid muscle and the trapezius muscle.
AREAS OF INFLUENCE	Sternocleidomastoid, trapezius, cervical spine, head, shoulder, scapula, thoracic vertebrae.
RELATIVE CONDITIONS	Shoulder pain, cervical pain, anxiety.

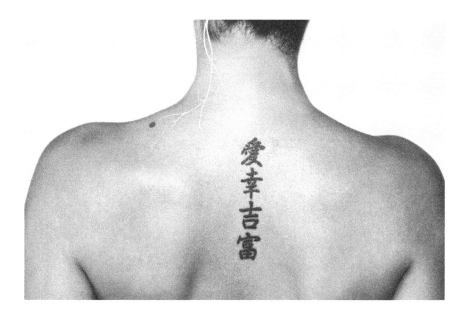

Figure 6.13 Spinal accessory Neuropuncture acupoint

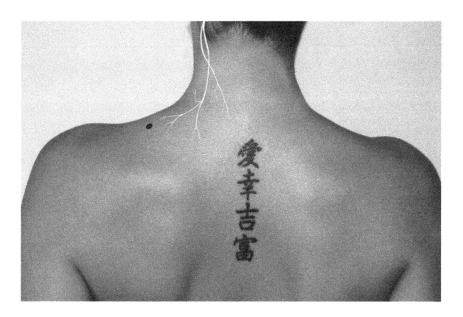

Figure 6.14 Spinal accessory nerves

Lateral antebrachial
Neuropuncture acupoint

TCM CLASSICAL ACUPUNCTURE POINT VICINITY	LI11–Qu Che.
SPINAL SEGMENT INNERVATION	c5, c6, c7.
AREAS OF INFLUENCE	Elbow, face, cervical spine, forearm, hand, shoulder.
RELATIVE CONDITIONS	Lateral epicondylitis, paresthesia, radiculopathy, headache, cervical pain.

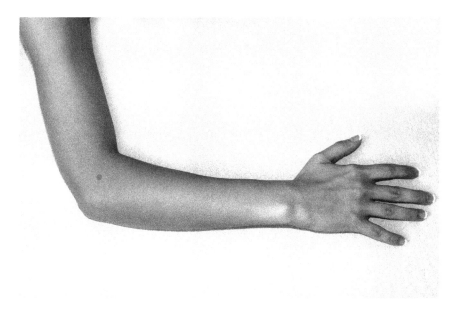

Figure 6.15 Lateral antebrachial Neuropuncture acupoint

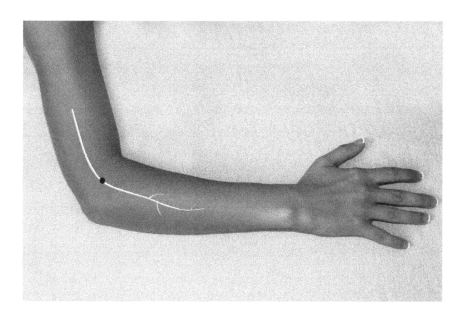

Figure 6.16 Lateral antebrachial nerves

Deep radial
Neuropuncture acupoint

TCM CLASSICAL ACUPUNCTURE POINT VICINITY	Distal/inferior to LI10.
SPINAL SEGMENT INNERVATION	c5, c6, c7, c8, t1. Posterior cord of the brachial plexus.
AREAS OF INFLUENCE	Forearm, hands, thumb/index, middle finger, biceps, shoulder/trap/scalenus/same side of face/ear/eye, cervical spine.
RELATIVE CONDITIONS	Lateral epicondylitis, cervical conditions, shoulder pain and frozen shoulder conditions, fibromyalgia syndrome. If "active" stage, needle for *any* pain syndrome, paresthesia, headaches.

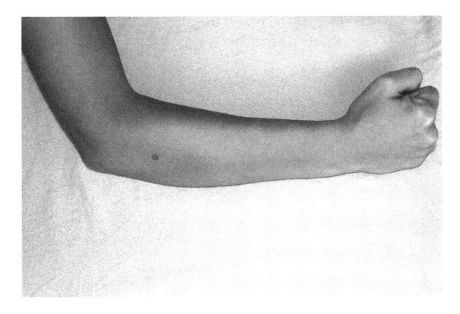

Figure 6.17 Deep radial Neuropuncture acupoint

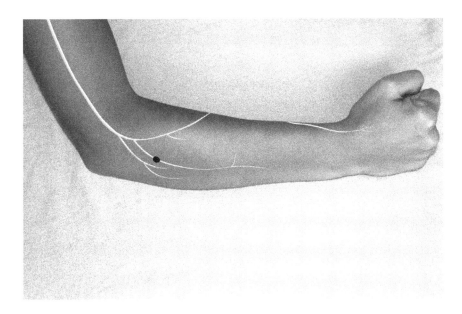

Figure 6.18 Deep radial nerves

Superficial radial
Neuropuncture acupoint

TCM CLASSICAL ACUPUNCTURE POINT VICINITY	LI4–He Gu.
SPINAL SEGMENT INNERVATION	c3, c4, c5, c6, c7, c8. Posterior cord of the brachial plexus.
AREAS OF INFLUENCE	Hand, forearm, elbow, shoulder, cervical spine, face, chest, stomach, hypothalamus, PAG.
RELATIVE CONDITIONS	Pain anywhere, especially same-side face, neck, throat. Cervical pathologies originating from c3–c8.

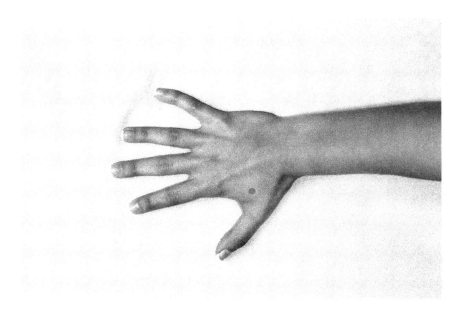

Figure 6.19 Superficial radial Neuropuncture acupoint

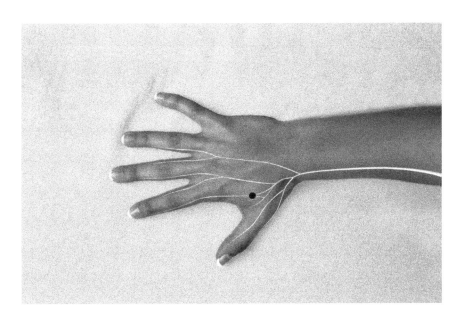

Figure 6.20 Superficial radial nerves

Deep median Neuropuncture acupoint

TCM CLASSICAL ACUPUNCTURE POINT VICINITY	PC6–Nei Guan.
SPINAL SEGMENT INNERVATION	C6, C7, C8, T1. Medial and lateral cord of the brachial plexus.
AREAS OF INFLUENCE	Carpal tunnel, fingers, hand, wrist, cardiac muscle.
RELATIVE CONDITIONS	Conditions treated: carpal tunnel, any median nerve pathology. Cervical conditions affecting C6–T1, hypertension.

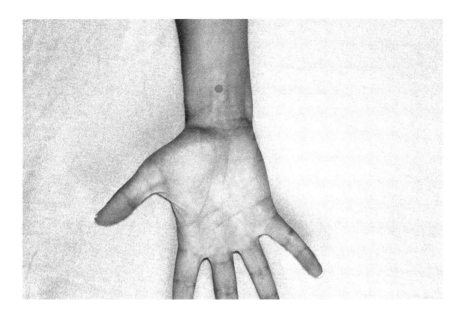

Figure 6.21 Deep median Neuropuncture acupoint

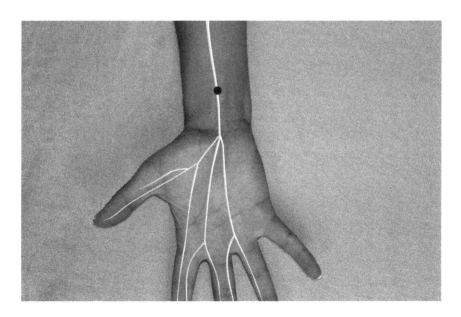

Figure 6.22 Deep median nerves

Ulnar
Neuropuncture acupoint

TCM CLASSICAL ACUPUNCTURE POINT VICINITY	Distal, but in the same groove, to HT7 (Shenmen)–HT5 (Tong Li).
SPINAL SEGMENT INNERVATION	c7, c8. Medial cord of the brachial plexus.
AREAS OF INFLUENCE	Wrist, fingers, arm, chest, cardiac muscle, reticular activating system of the brain.
RELATIVE CONDITIONS	Neural-associated conditions, insomnia, emotional instability, anxiety, cervical pain, neck and shoulder pain, upper back pain, same-sided weakness.

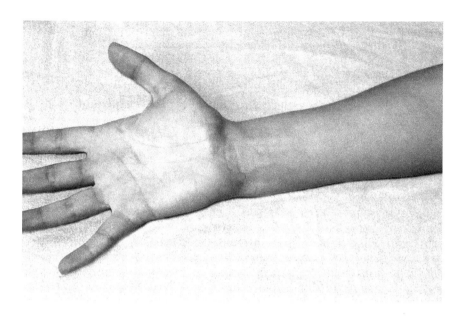

Figure 6.23 Ulnar Neuropuncture acupoint

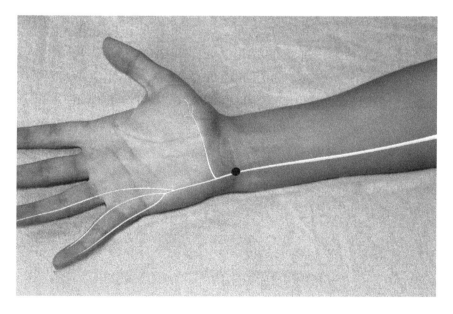

Figure 6.24 Ulnar nerves

Carpal tunnel release
Neuropuncture acupoint

TCM CLASSICAL ACUPUNCTURE POINT VICINITY	Proximal to PC8–Long Gong.
AREAS OF INFLUENCE	Hand, carpal tunnel, palmar side, fingers.
RELATIVE CONDITIONS	Carpal tunnel syndrome, hand pain, wrist pain.

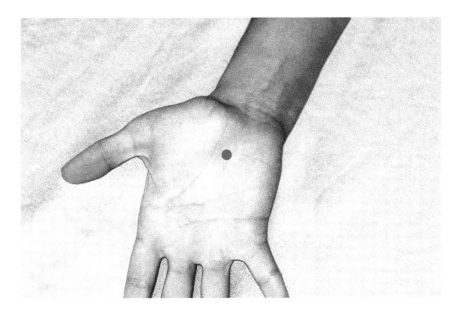

Figure 6.25 Carpal tunnel release Neuropuncture acupoint

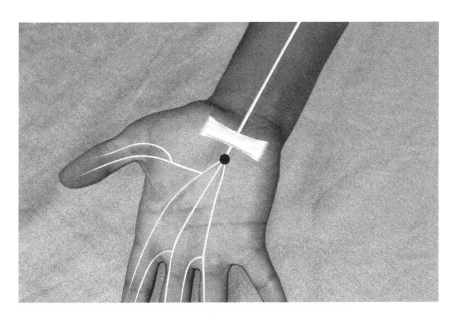

Figure 6.26 Carpal tunnel release nerves

Saphenous
Neuropuncture acupoint

TCM CLASSICAL ACUPUNCTURE POINT VICINITY	SP9.
SPINAL SEGMENT INNERVATION	L2, L3, L4. Extension of the femoral nerve–lumbar plexus L2–4.
AREAS OF INFLUENCE	Knee, foot, groin, abdominal cavity, lumbar spine.
RELATIVE CONDITIONS	Lower back pain, paresthesia, lower abdomen pathologies, urogenital pathologies, renal conditions, impotence, leg pain and weakness.

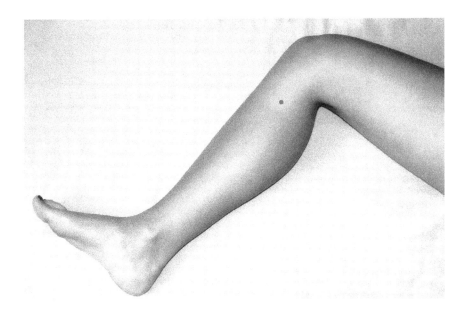

Figure 6.27 Saphenous Neuropuncture acupoint

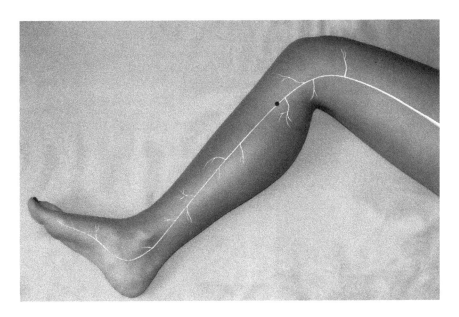

Figure 6.28 Saphenous nerves

Tibial
Neuropuncture acupoint

TCM CLASSICAL ACUPUNCTURE POINT VICINITY	SP6–San Yin Jiao.
SPINAL SEGMENT INNERVATION	L4, L5, S1, S2, S3. Branch of sciatic nerve.
AREAS OF INFLUENCE	Inner lower leg, sole of foot, groin, abdomen, reproductive organs.
RELATIVE CONDITIONS	Sciatica, paresthesia, plantar, fasciitis, lower abdomen pathologies, obstetric and gynecological pathologies.

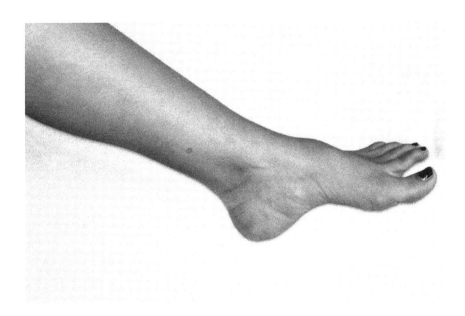

Figure 6.29 Tibial Neuropuncture acupoint

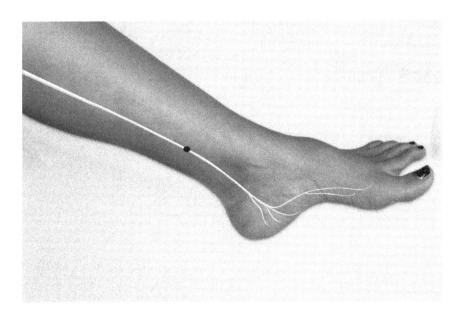

Figure 6.30 Tibial nerves

Common peroneal[1]
Neuropuncture acupoint

TCM CLASSICAL ACUPUNCTURE POINT VICINITY	Superior and posterior to GB34. Posterior to the fibular head.
BRANCH NERVE	Bifurcation of sciatic nerve.
SPINAL SEGMENT INNERVATION	L5, S1, S2, S3.
AREAS OF INFLUENCE	Calf, lumbar spine, lumbar muscles, knee, reproductive organs.
RELATIVE CONDITIONS	Sciatica, paresthesia, lower back pain, lower leg pathologies.

---

1   This nerve runs directly along the posterior border of the fibular head.

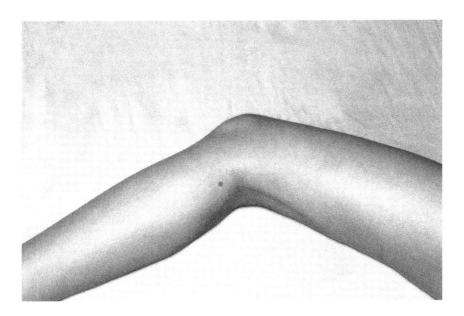

Figure 6.31 Common peroneal Neuropuncture acupoint

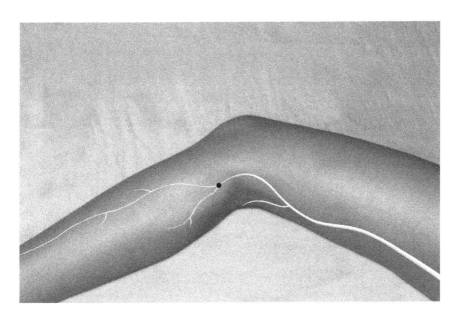

Figure 6.32 Common peroneal nerves

Sural
Neuropuncture acupoint

TCM CLASSICAL ACUPUNCTURE POINT VICINITY	BL57.
BRANCH NERVE	Branch of the tibial nerve.
SPINAL SEGMENT INNERVATION	L2–L4.
AREAS OF INFLUENCE	Calf, Achilles tendon, knee, lateral aspect of foot, little toe.
RELATIVE CONDITIONS	Calf pain, hemorrhoids, radiculopathy of the leg, paresthesia of the lower leg, lumbar pain.

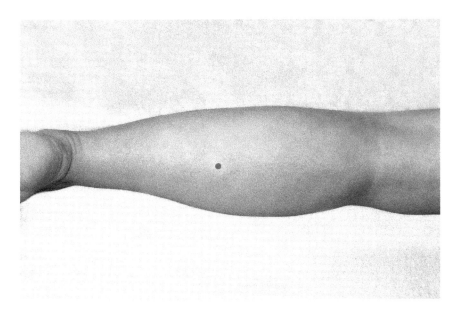

Figure 6.33 Sural Neuropuncture acupoint

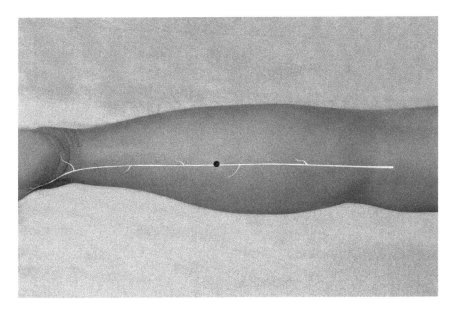

Figure 6.34 Sural nerves

Medial popliteal
Neuropuncture acupoint

TCM CLASSICAL ACUPUNCTURE POINT VICINITY	BL40.
BRANCH NERVES	Common fibular and the tibial branch.
SPINAL SEGMENT INNERVATION	L4–S3.
AREAS OF INFLUENCE	Knee, lumbar spine, calf.
RELATIVE CONDITIONS	Lumbar pain, sciatica, knee pain, rhematoid arthritis, calf and hamstring pathologies.

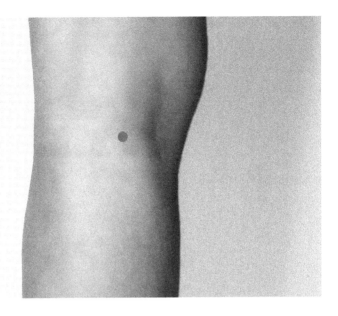

Figure 6.35 Medial popliteal Neuropuncture acupoint

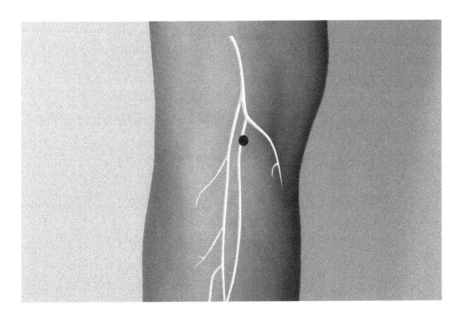

Figure 6.36 Medial popliteal nerves

Deep peroneal
Neuropuncture acupoint

TCM CLASSICAL ACUPUNCTURE POINT VICINITY	LV3–Tai Chong.
SPINAL SEGMENT INNERVATION	L4–S2, distal branch of the sciatica nerve. Also referred to as the fibular nerve.
AREAS OF INFLUENCE	Foot, calf, knee, leg, low back, lower abdomen, reproductive organs, pituitary, hypothalamus.
RELATIVE CONDITIONS	Sciatica, paresthesia, neuralgia, from low back pain to foot pain to big toe pain, obstetric and gynecological conditions, headaches, migraines, generalized body pain, fibromyalgia syndrome.

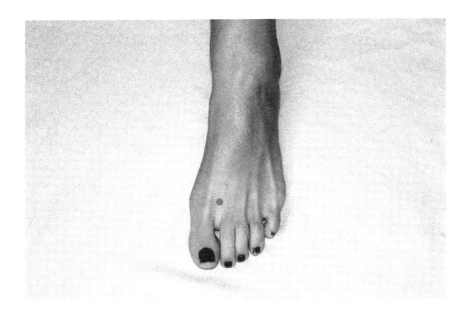

Figure 6.37 Deep peroneal Neuropuncture acupoint

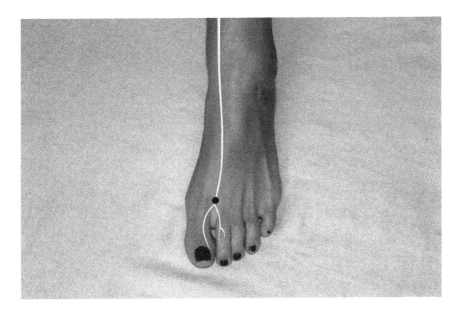

Figure 6.38 Deep peroneal Neuropuncture nerves

Posterior superior iliac spine (PSIS) Neuropuncture acupoint

TCM CLASSICAL ACUPUNCTURE POINT VICINITY	Regional to Yao Yan.
SPINAL SEGMENT INNERVATION	L2–L5, superior cluneal nerves.
AREAS OF INFLUENCE	Low back, sacral crest, lumbar spine.
RELATIVE CONDITIONS	Sciatica, sacral pain, obstetric and gynecological pain, lumbar conditions, renal conditions, urogenital conditions.

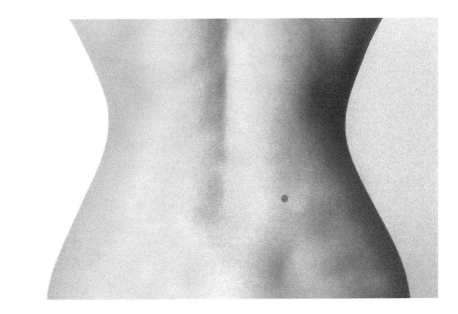

Figure 6.39 Posterior superior iliac spine Neuropuncture acupoint

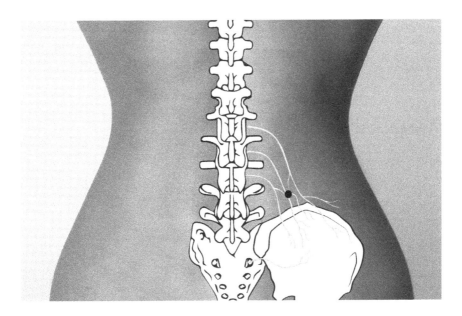

Figure 6.40 Posterior superior iliac spine nerves

Paraspinal
Neuropuncture acupoint

TCM CLASSICAL ACUPUNCTURE POINT VICINITY	TCM Back Shu.
SPINAL SEGMENT INNERVATION	Associated parallel vertebral segment.
AREAS OF INFLUENCE	Affiliated visceral innervations. Level with spinal segment.
RELATIVE CONDITIONS	Associated visceral pathology, local neuromuscular conditions.

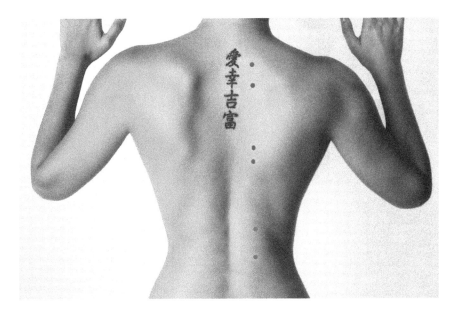

Figure 6.41 Paraspinal Neuropuncture acupoints

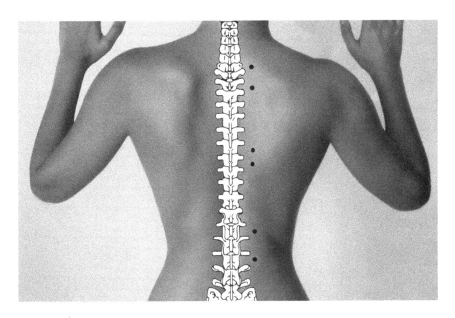

Figure 6.42 Parallel vertebral segmental bodies

Chapter 7

Explanation of Theory and the Clinical Application of Neuropuncture

Our body is the most powerful manufacturer of natural pharmaceutical drugs, homeostatic neuropeptides and healing biochemicals in the world, and we need to find a way to access these natural physiological processes. Research shows that the human body, particularly the human brain, when given the correct stimulation in the right environment, can produce practically any compound necessary for healing (Frisaldi, Piedimonte & Benedetti, 2015). Placebos have clearly illustrated this notion. Masters of meditation have been able to produce special immunoglobulins under deep meditation (Fernandes, Nóbrega & Tosta, 2012).

I have personally analyzed the specific neurophysiological process of acupuncture and research into the neuroscience of specific acupuncture protocols, and put it into a highly effective and reproducible system of treatment. When applying Neuropuncture to a medical case, you *must* apply a special mindset. It will take some time to adjust from the classical TCM energetic viewpoint to the neuroanatomy viewpoint, but what you will find is a concise, reproducible, exciting approach to treating patients. If your back studies are in TCM and classical acupuncture, trust me, it may be a difficult transition—*but* well worth it! You can still practice classical TCM with the addition of being aware and applying this information to the actual location and neurophysiological matrix of an acupuncture acupoint.

First determine the targeted neural-complex structures of the pathological condition, then choose the Neuropuncture acupoints that you want to stimulate to affect the pathological neurostructures or produce and release specific biochemicals. You can also employ any of the five neurophysiological mechanisms described in Chapter 4 and even combine several of them at once to really amplify the healing force. Applying the Neuropuncture theory of needling in several ways can include the following.

The five Neuropuncture treatment principles (NTPs)

The five NTPs are designed to apply the five neurophysiological mechanisms clinically to medical cases. Through understanding the mechanisms of how acupuncture works, the true pathways of electrical transmission, you can apply the treatment principles to your cases to focus that electrical transmission properly and with intent.

1. Focus on harnessing the "local effect."

2. Target a specific nerve (e.g. median, sciatica, facial).

3. Target a specific neural plexus. The idea is to stimulate a distal branch nerve that innervates the targeted nerve or neuro-complex.

4. Target a specific segment of the spine.

5. Target the CNS. Focus on specific receptors or areas of the brain.

Table 7.1 The five Neurophysiological mechanisms, five NTPS, and four EN treatment principles

Neurophysiological mechanisms	Neuropuncture treatment principles
1. Local effect	1. Harness local effect
2. Spinal segmental	2. Target specific nerve
3. EOC	3. Target specific neural plexus
4. CNS	4. Target specific spinal segment
5. Neuromuscular	5. Target CNS (release of specific neuropeptides)

Electrical Neuropuncture treatment principles

1. Reduce inflammation and begin repair of soft tissues, vs. strengthening soft tissues.
2. Targeting specific receptors for specific neuropeptide release.
3. Interrupt visceral dysfunctional autonomic reflexes.
4. Depolarize specific nerve pathways.

Understanding the NTPs then, after you have determined which neural tract is pathological (e.g. median nerve in carpal tunnel syndrome) or where the pathology exists neuroanatomically (e.g. herniated nucleus prolapse at L4/L5), and which tract can be targeted to be stimulated, choose the specific Neuropuncture acupoint that will accomplish the task. Below are examples of how to apply the NTPs:

NTP 1: Use local needling into, or on the border of, the site of trauma, pathology, and local infections. Use general local needling, superficial or deep, and "osteopuncture" (see later in this chapter) for accessible bone pain/arthritis and tendinitis. This NTP has been used for simple conditions, from swollen inflamed joints, sinus infections, and stubborn non-healing surgical incisions, to skin infections or burns.

NTP 2: After determining the root pathological nerve, you can needle distal, "above and below," Neuropuncture points to affect that connected pathological nerve. A great example is carpal tunnel syndrome. Needling the carpal tunnel release Neuropuncture point and then needling the median Neuropuncture point, and running 25 HZ microcurrent through those points directly targets the median nerve and the carpal tunnel. Another few examples are the trigeminal nerve for trigeminal neuralgia, or the facial nerve for Bell's palsy.

NTP 3: Sometimes you may come across a nerve that is pathological but you cannot directly access that nerve root. So, determine what nerve, distally, you can stimulate that runs up and into the same neural plexus that will affect the pathological nerve. The pudendal nerve is a great example. I will use the tibial Neuropuncture point (SP6), to access the sacral plexus and affect the pudendal nerve indirectly. Another example is the sciatic nerve, and needling the common peroneal nerve, a distal bifurcation of the sciatic nerve.

NTP 4: First determine the exact spinal segment that you need to target. You can use the dermatome and visceral charts (Tables 2.2 and 2.3) at the beginning of the book for easy reference. Then needle motor points or Neuropuncture acupoints that innervate the desired spinal segment and EN them. Using MRI imaging can determine the exact level of disc pathology, and if you are focusing on organ health the visceral tomes must be used for accurate, focused treatment.

NTP 5: This NTP is knowing how and when we apply the specific frequencies to target and release specific neuropeptides. In this NTP we are focusing on the stimulation directly to the CNS, the most powerful producer of neurochemicals in the world.

Utilizing specific electrical frequencies on specific Neuropuncture points focuses your treatment in a very special way. A great example of this is with Parkinson's—by needling the Neuropuncture protocol we are targeting the tyrosine hydroxylase enzyme and also issuing a neuroprotective property to the brain itself. All of this is being completed utilizing specific electrical frequencies on specific points. Another simple example is targeting any of the three endorphins with specific electrical frequencies.

Once you have determined which neural tract is pathological (e.g. median nerve in carpal tunnel syndrome) or where the pathology exists neuroanatomically (e.g. herniated nucleus prolapse at L4/ L5), and which tract can be targeted to be stimulated, choose the specific Neuropuncture acupoint that will accomplish the task. Below are examples of applying the neurophysical mechanisms of acupuncture to clinical treatments.

- Mechanism 1: Use local needling into, or on the border of, the site of trauma, pathology, and local infections. Use general local needling and osteopuncture (see later in the chapter) for accessible bone pain/arthritis and tendinitis.

- Mechanism 2: After determining the root pathological nerve, you can needle distal Neuropuncture acupoints to affect that connected pathological nerve.

- Mechanism 3: Access these spinal segments by needling large muscle groups whose motor nerve innervates that targeted spinal segment. You can also needle the Neuropuncture acupoints that innervate the targeted nerve plexus directly, and both approaches will affect the associated viscera (protocols are in Chapter 8).

- Mechanism 4: For a general systemic effect, needle bilateral points or ipsilateral ones (i.e. superficial radial nerve, deep peroneal nerve, tibial nerve). Usually, two limb

Neuropuncture acupoints, bilateral ones, are needled and EA applied so that the muscle contraction is visible and a nice De Qi sensation is produced (protocols are in Chapter 8). This will ensure the maximum release of endorphins for systemic pain relief. Auricular EA can be applied to enhance the effect.

Below is an example of combining several of the NTPs for a sciatica case:

1. Local needling: HTJJ L3–L5/S1.

2. Distal needling: Common peroneal Neuropuncture acupoint and saphenous Neuropuncture acupoint.

3. Then apply EA: 2–100 HZ millicurrent to target the mu and delta receptors for the release of beta-endorphins, enkephalins, and dynorphins. It has been shown that burst stimulation results in the largest release of neuropeptides. In this example you are directly depolarizing the sciatic nerve and stimulating the maximum cerebral release of endorphins (Filshie & White, 1998).

Also, remember that in applying this new treatment it is effective to take another, different look at diagnosis and pathophysiology. Nowadays, with an accurate Western medical diagnosis, we can modify very specific neural tracts and target receptors to influence physiology.

Assessment utilizing a 1–4 Pain Upon Palpation (PUP) scale

Dissecting an acupuncture point's anatomy and physiology shows us that the location of classical acupuncture points consists of a unique neural matrix network, lying under the surface of the skin.

Research has examined acupuncture points thoroughly and has concluded that a "functional" acupuncture point is the specific area where bone, muscle, nerve, fascia, and skin conjugate. It is here that neurovascular bundles and connective tissue contain abundant nerves and blood vessels. It is also here that these acupoints have the nodes and terminal ends where the classical Zang-Fu organs, meridians, Qi, and blood were thought to infuse at the body's surface. I have always applied the PUP scale for assessing a patient's pain. Applying that PUP scale to Neuropuncture acupoints is a simple way to assess the state of the point.

The PUP scale is a simple way of locating your Neuropuncture acupoint of choice before needling. The practitioner utilizes a 2 lb of pressure scale and a clinical PUP scale of 1–4. When applied to the location of interest, it is a simple clinical way of determining the proper location and status of the Neuropuncture acupoint. You want to target the nerve by trapping it between the bone, or between your fingers gripping the muscle, and eliciting a sensory response from the patient. In doing this, you can determine the phase that the Neuropuncture point is in, as well as the location to needle. I personally assess it by how much neural inflammation is present. Based on the pain scale throughout the entire assessment, you can incorporate dietary recommendations—alkaline vs. basic diet—EPA/DHA dosage, and so on.

You may ask yourself: "How do I measure 2 lb of pressure?" What I did for a while was this: Whenever I was in the grocery section of the food store I would use my index and middle fingers and apply 2 lb of pressure on the produce scale. After a while, I became familiar with the proper amount of pressure to apply. Remember that this is the pressure applied directly to the nerve, and in some cases pressure is applied against the bone. It is a subjective measure—and I really try to avoid subjective techniques—but after training your sensitivity skills, it becomes quite accurate.

Utilizing a 1–4 PUP scale:

  1 = light, barely noticeable

  2 = moderately bothersome

  3 = very uncomfortable

  4 = patient jerks away from pressure with facial and possibly
       vocal display of discomfort.

After reviewing the pathological neuropathology of your patient's chief complaint, next begin to assess the Neuropuncture acupoints in referencing and applying the five NTPs (see earlier).

What remains is the construction of your protocol from your assessment. While assessing Neuropuncture acupoints, apply pressure to the points and observe the patient's reaction (see Table 7.2; a scale of 0 would be no reaction, indicating a latent phase).

Table 7.2 Pain Upon Palpation (PUP) scale

Scale number 1 (latent phase)	Light, barely noticeable.
Scale number 2 (passive phase)	Moderate, bothersome.
Scale number 3 (initial active phase)	Very uncomfortable.
Scale number 4 (full active phase)	Patient jerks away from pressure with facial and possibly vocal display of discomfort.

Neuropuncture acupoint assessment

The latent phase (scale number 1) is when a 2 lb pressure is applied to the Neuropuncture acupoint and there is no reaction from the patient. For comparison, in the passive phase with 2 lb of pressure, there is a perception of discomfort by the patient but nothing on a grand scale. In the latent phase there is no reason to needle these

Neuropuncture acupoints unless you are applying one of the five NTPs accordingly.

The passive phase (scale number 2) is when 2 lb of pressure is applied to the Neuropuncture acupoint and there is an obvious sensation of discomfort reported by the patient, but no physical pulling away. The patient may say: "Yes, I feel that but there is not too much pain." This indicates the level of neural inflammation and that this specific Neuropuncture acupoint needs to be needled. Remember, the first Neuropuncture mechanism illustrates the effects of local needling.

The initial active phase (scale number 3) is when with 2 lb of pressure applied the patient feels very uncomfortable and reports a feeling of pain. These Neuropuncture acupoints are excellent to needle due to the fact that they will enter the fully active phase if not treated.

The full active phase (scale number 4) is when without any pressure the Neuropuncture acupoint is in a constant state of pain. These Neuropuncture acupoints need to be needled, and the sensitivity only confirms, and diagnostically illustrates, the necessity of needling these Neuropuncture acupoints in systemic pain cases such as fibromyalgia syndrome.

So, utilizing this scale, if a particular Neuropuncture acupoint is in the passive phase, it can still be needled but may not have a great amount of inflammation in that area. You would needle a passive phase Neuropuncture acupoint if it was dependent on the five NTPs being applied. If a Neuropuncture acupoint is in the active phase, then you should definitely consider needling and properly stimulating it. You can use this assessment scale to give you a preliminary scan of your patient's potential Neuropuncture acupoint status and overall neural health. I find this palpation assessment to be very useful in chronic pain cases.

Needle technique

Remember that you do not needle directly into the nerve itself! When you insert the needle and guide it along the targeted nerve root or at the targeted nerve, it is important to understand that you stop just above or in front of any large nerve roots (the aim is to stimulate the underlying delta fibers). Remember to ask for feedback from the patient. You know you have hit your mark when the patient feels the stimulation (i.e. the afferent fibers have been stimulated). Be sure not to directly puncture the nerve! You need to be gentle and mindful while needling. Make sure your patient reports a De Qi comfortable sensation after needle stimulation. An achy, sore, deep muscle ache or distension are all excellent signs. A sharp or very uncomfortable sensation comes from the C-fiber, which you do not want to stimulate. If at the time of insertion your patient feels a sharp, painful sensation, just remove the needle, relocate the acupoint and re-needle. Sometimes that initial painful sensation is felt by the patient due to a local hair follicle or a small C-fiber accidently being hit.

You can utilize any of the classical needle techniques: lift and thrust, wagging the blue green dragon's tail, siphoning, and twirl. If you get a local muscle fasciculation, that's great; and if your patient at first feels a "prick," that is fine, as long as the prick sensation does not continue. Warmth and coolness are also acceptable. You *do not* want any strong, painful, stabbing, excessively sharp or burning sensations. Again, this guidance coincides with that found in the TCM classics.

Needle properly, in a non-aggressive manner. Due to the manufactured structural design of an acupuncture needle, it is difficult to cause serious tissue damage. However, you must approach with "cautioned confidence." It is important to know about anatomy and, in particular, the specific neuroanatomy underlying the Neuropuncture point—or, for that matter, *any* acupuncture acupoint that you tend to needle. Remember that the classic TCM acupoints are fantastic areas to examine for the underlying neurophysiology. The technique for needling Neuropuncture acupoints that may be sensitive or lie in congested areas is to gently lift the skin and needle perpendicularly. Once the needle is inserted, slide the needle between the layers of tissue and then release the skin and allow the connective tissue to gently pull the needle into the point. You can further stimulate gently to obtain De Qi.

The acupuncture needle can be inserted utilizing traditional hand insertion or guide-tube insertion. If utilizing hand insertion, make sure to grip the needle firmly to support the shaft while inserting the needle. In either technique, the needle, after insertion, must be stimulated until the patient feels a De Qi sensation. Remember, a comfortable Qi sensation is propagated, not a sharp, stabbing, or burning painful sensation. A desired sensation is one of a dull muscle ache, a sore-achy sensation, warmness, heaviness, distension, gentle traveling, fullness, or even a small muscle fasciculation. As explained above, these classical sensations are the small delta, peripheral, and afferent nerve fibers firing and eventually hitting their mark, targeting a nerve tract or specific areas of the brain. When you apply electricity to the point, as in EA, again it still must produce a nice achy, dull, sore sensation to maximize the benefits.

When it comes to the size and gauge of needles, I sometimes like to use 0.5 x 20 gauge needles. These are very tiny, so they are not used for large neuromuscular points; the superficial nerves have been shown to affect the larger nerve tracts. But, with thicker muscle layers and denser tissue, longer and thicker gauged needles are needed. The needle gauge used depends on the patient's body type and size, as well as the Neuropuncture acupoint under assessment.

Osteopuncture

In this technique, you needle directly into the periosteum of the bone. You do not needle deeply though. It is effective to just insert the needle with a guide tube just above the targeted bone and tap several needles into the bone gently. This is a great way to treat most orthopedic bone conditions, ligament issues, and any stubborn fractures that have periosteum access.

Electro-Neuropuncture (EN)

This is the application of electricity through the Neuropuncture acupoints at specific frequencies, for specific intervals of time, for the purpose of targeting specific neuro-tissue (e.g. receptors, areas of the brain). EA applied to the referenced Neuropuncture acupoints can maximize the desired effect and allow us to measure closely the exact amount of stimulation for reproducible outcomes. Remember, in the 1950s EA was used in China to replace manual stimulation for doctors. This has led to an application of protocols that are reproducible and measurable. In many cases, you can add some form of electricity—millicurrent, microcurrent, piezo, pachipachi—to maximize the benefits of treatment.

Always be careful in choosing which current. You do not want to aggravate the condition with excessive or too powerful stimulation at the wrong time of the treatment plan. When applied correctly, this will help to stimulate the Neuropuncture acupoints, and when applied appropriately it enhances the outcome by stimulating the neuropathways in a controlled, focused, homeostatic way. It is important to use EA as a tool to target a focused electrical current. In this way, the intensity does not have to always be a comfortable, strong sensation; it can be just barely perceivable.

It is also common for the muscles innervated by the nerve to contract, fasciculate, and "jump" to the frequency. That is ideal! Just be sure that your patient is comfortable. In most of my treatments I have my patients "dancing." I have had very few complaints and the outcomes are highly effective. For example, while treating migraines, if you are applying EA to the superficial radial Neuropuncture acupoint or to the greater auricular Neuropuncture acupoint, and the superficial radial Neuropuncture acupoint begins to "tap" to the frequency, then that is ideal. Similarly in the treatment of sciatica, if the common peroneal Neuropuncture acupoint begins to "jump" to the frequency, then again that will yield the desired outcome.

Table 7.3 is a reference chart of the electrical acupuncture protocols for targeting receptors in the endorphin system for maximum pain relief.

Table 7.3 EA protocols for targeting receptors

Neuropeptide	Receptor	Frequency/amperage	Location
Beta-endorphins	Mu/delta	2–4 HZ millicurrent	Midbrain/PAG/pituitary
Enkephalins	Mu/delta	2–4 HZ millicurrent	Dorsal horn of spinal cord
Dynorphins	Kappa	50–100 HZ millicurrent	Brainstem/spine
5-HTP	5-HTP receptor	20–50 HZ millicurrent	CNS
Oxytocin	–	15–30 HZ millicurrent Max HZ 2–30 millicurrent	CNS

Clinically, when I have applied EA to my Neuropuncture protocol, I have found it to be effective to begin with microcurrent and then slowly change to millicurrent. There are several reasons for this—for starters, microcurrent has been proven scientifically to help to reduce inflammation, stimulate cellular respiration via increased ATP production and help to repair tissue damage (Cheng *et al.*, 1982). Millicurrent is what has been mainly used throughout the scientific community in clinical trials and has been shown to strengthen tissues, break up adhesions and be highly effective in targeting the release of specific neuropeptides.

Table 7.4 is an example of a treatment protocol utilizing EN.[1] Remember it is always important to adjust your treatments according to your clinical assessment.

Table 7.4 Electro-Neuropuncture treatment protocol

Treatment	Frequency/amperage	Duration
1st treatment	25 HZ microcurrent	25–30 min
2nd to 3rd treatment	Single stimulation 2 HZ millicurrent	25–30 min
4th to 5th treatment	Burst stimulation 2–15 HZ mixed millicurrent	25–30 min
6th to 8th treatment	Burst stimulation 2–100 HZ mixed millicurrent	25–30 min

---

1   For more information on needling techniques and video demonstrations, visit www.neuropuncture.org.

Chapter 8

Neuropuncture Treatment Protocols

Three extra Neuropuncture points

The following Neuropuncture acupoints are additional to the original set. These are either new acupuncture points altogether or traditional acupuncture points that are regularly found in research and therefore it is important to know the neuroanatomy of these points. They are also common points that I use, and I focus on the underlying network of physical structures, not necessarily an "energetic" location.

Anterior tibialis motor Neuropuncture point (ATNP)

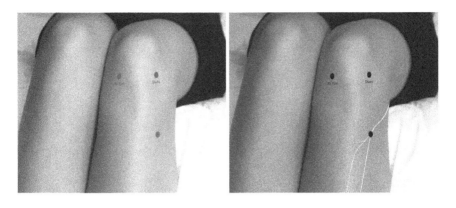

Figure 8.1 Anterior tibialis Neuropuncture acupoint (ST36)

Figure 8.2 Anterior tibialis nerves

Philtrum Neuropuncture point (PhNP)

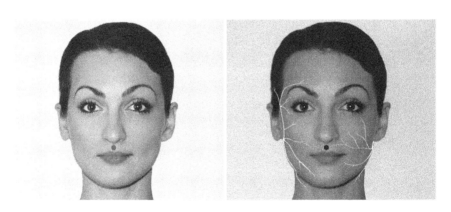

Figure 8.3 Philtrum Neuropuncture acupoint (DU26)

Figure 8.4 Philtrum nerves

Auricular posterior Neuropuncture point (APNP)

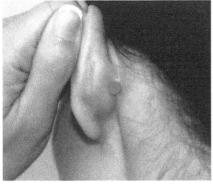 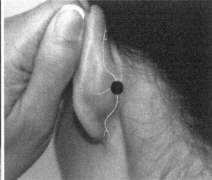

Figure 8.5 Auricular posterior Neuropuncture acupoint

Figure 8.6 Auricular posterior nerves

Before we continue, there are some additional abbreviations that you should be aware of:

Electro-Acupuncture (EA): If this appears after a point prescription, it implies that the group of acupuncture points just prior to the symbol, EA, is attached with a single lead. If using a Pantheon EA stimulator, then the specificity of the placement of the red and black leads is insignificant. I generally place my red lead on the points closer to the heart and the black lead closer to any distal points, mainly for aesthetic purposes.

Acupuncture motor point (MP): Usually you will see this just after the name of a specific large muscle, indicating that the motor point of that said muscle is to be needled.

Electro-Neuropuncture protocols

All of the following protocols are ones that I use regularly with amazing success. I firmly believe that you can trust these protocols as I consistently receive positive feedback from practitioners from all around the world. They are a combination of published research that I have reviewed, my own clinical application, and the application of the evidence-based neurophysiology of the condition to the neurophysiology of EA.

If the protocol is taken from published research, then the research was done on humans and I have read about it in several publications, not just one, though there may have been some slight alterations to the protocol. Most of this research was completed in the USA at universities or research hospitals, and concurrent research has been found in research medical journals from China, Germany, the Czech Republic, and India. Just as in any acupuncture protocol, you must look at every case individually and make any adjustments that you see fit. That is what I term the "acupuncture dosage": the needle retention time interval, frequency of electrical wave, the current of the electrical stimulation, and any needle adjustments needed.

Adding auricular or scalp acupuncture points, or a point for pulse or tongue findings, are always encouraged. I personally use TCM tongue and TCM pulse diagnosis very regularly, though more so for my patient's herbal prescriptions and diet recommendations.

Please keep in mind that the level of intensity of stimulation should always be appropriate to the case and patient. "Comfortably strong" is what we are looking for. It is not a pain tolerance test! I think of this as the De Qi of EA. As mentioned throughout this book, the EA De Qi should be gentle and warming, it can have distension or fullness, it can be strong at times, dull, or achy—these sensations are all fine. What we don't want is for the EA De Qi to be burning, painful, or stabbing, or uncomfortable in any other way. Sometimes 25 HZ microcurrent is the best for a gentle stimulation to balance the nervous system and promote healing. Below I have listed the protocol using abbreviations, the placement of the leads for EA, commentary on the placement of EA leads, and small explanation. I use Pantheon machines because they are FDA approved and offer millicurrent *and* microcurrent. Since the waveform of the Pantheon is bi-phasic, I am not concerned with where the red or black lead goes. For aesthetics I normally place the black lead distal and the red lead closer to the heart. Just be sure that you have the lead in the correct current plug-in. Enjoy!

Note: The Neuropuncture acupoint prescription column shows exactly how I document the prescriptions in my treatment notes at work in my EHR.

Table 8.1 Neuropuncture protocols for common conditions

Disease/ condition	Neuropuncture acupoint prescription	EA placement explanation	Neuropuncture dosage	Commentary
Alzheimer's/ Dementia	DU20–Yintang: EA, Si Shen Cong–Anmien: EA	For this protocol I have the patient lie prone (face down) on the treatment table for easy access to the scalp points and adjust the headrest so that Yintang is accessible. Another position is to needle Anmien, then guide the patient down onto their back in a supine position. Use one lead to attach Yintang to DU20 (Pai Hui), then use another lead to attach the right Si Shen Cong to the right Anmien acupoint, then the last lead to attach the left Si Shen Cong to the left Anmien acupoint. Remember to set the dial to "mixed" frequency to 2–5 HZ millicurrent. I combine this with the *Neuropuncture Parkinson's protocol* using a separate Pantheon, to maximize the neuroprotective properties.	EA: 2–5 HZ for 30 minutes. 2 times a week for 6 weeks = 12 sessions. 3 times a week for 4 weeks = 12 sessions.	Research has shown that this helps to reduce beta-amyloid sheets.

Anxiety	NADA (Shenmen)–Tranquilizer/MO: EA Acute and right-sided pulse is weak *add*: ST36(B): EA Chronic and (L) pulse is deep and xu *add*: TNP: EA	Whenever I needle NADA, I use the dominant side ear. So, in this case you would needle Shenmen, from the NADA protocol on the dominant side, and then connect the opposite lead to Tranquilizer/Master Oscillator (MO) in the opposite ear. Thread into and along the tragus to connect one needle to the Tranquilizer and MO point.	EA: 2 HZ millicurrent for 25–45 minutes. 2 times a week for 6 weeks = 12 sessions. 3 times a week for 4 weeks = 12 sessions.	I really enjoy using this protocol for opioid detox withdrawal induced anxiety. This has a powerful effect on calming the patient down and lasts for a good 24 hours. So, with opioid withdrawal anxiety I treat the patient daily for the first week.
Cerebral Vascular Accident (CVA) stroke with unilateral paralysis	Opposite the paralysis Scalp Motor associated areas—Neuropuncture acupoints on affected limbs.	Here you insert several needles along, and within, the Scalp Motor area associated with the symptoms opposite the paralysis. Then clip a few of the scalp needles together with an alligator clip and attach the other lead to the opposite side associated Neuropuncture acupoint on the affected paralyzed limb.	EA: 2 HZ millicurrent for 25 minutes. Every other day in the beginning weeks, 1–2 times a day.	Although I do not have published research to support this protocol, the neuroanatomy application and similar protocols that I have researched support my experience that this can reduce cerebral lesions—the electrical stimulation directly traces out the pathway that is affected. Rehab is also extremely important in helping to connect the neural pathways.

Disease/ condition	Neuropuncture acupoint prescription	EA placement explanation	Neuropuncture dosage	Commentary
Carpal tunnel syndrome	MNP–CRTNP: EA	When I insert a needle into CRTNP, I either firmly grip the patient's wrist, as a distraction and to suppress some nerve firing, or have them cough on the count of 3. On 3, tap the needle in quickly. Then, once it is inserted, I apply a little firm pressure on the wrist as I slowly insert the needle deeper into the desired depth. Then I attach one lead to the CRTNP and the opposite lead to the MNP. When you increase the intensity on this protocol, you should adjust it really slowly as this area can be sensitive. You can always add SRNP to LANP, in the same way, for a more chronic and severe case.	EA: 25 HZ microcurrent for 20 minutes. 2 times a week for 6 weeks = 12 sessions. 3 times a week for 4 weeks = 12 sessions.	This protocol will target the median nerve and the carpal tunnel directly. Utilizing the 25 HZ microcurrent aids in reducing inflammation and repairing soft tissue.

| Dental analgesia | SRNP(B): EA
You can also add ST6: EA | Wait for a dull, achy sensation at SRNP. I personally used this protocol, without ST6, for a mercury filling removal (and a second tooth was drilled out). I used no medication, just Neuropuncture.

I have a video clip of a doctor of dental sciences (DDS) wearing a mask in the middle of the procedure. She is turning towards the camera and stating she cannot believe that I am not feeling the procedure! You can see it on my website: www.Neuropuncture.org | EA: 2–30 HZ millicurrent for 20+ minutes. | This protocol is an example of applying the neuroanatomy of the acupuncture point and knowing its termination.

SRNP sends a signal along the radial nerve that then connects with the brachial plexus and then into the spinal cord and up to the brain. In the brain it has ends that terminate in the hypothalamus and at 2 HZ you will be activating the PAG through the release of beta-endorphins.

Also remember the spinal segment mechanism, and how at the level of the dorsal horn there are three neuropeptides that get released. |

Disease/ condition	Neuropuncture acupoint prescription	EA placement explanation	Neuropuncture dosage	Commentary
Depression	DU20–Yintang: EA, TNP(B): EA	Simply attach the red clip to Yintang and the black clip to DU20 (Pai Hui), using one lead. Then you attach the right tibial Neuropuncture point (TNP) (SP6) to the left TNP (SP6) with one lead.	EA: 2 HZ millicurrent for 25 minutes. 2 times a week for 6 weeks = 12 sessions. 3 times a week for 4 weeks = 12 sessions.	I have seen this protocol many times in publications and they always state how it is effective on the metabolism of medication, specifically Prozac (it targets the D1 prefrontal dopamine receptors). I have added the TNP aspect for energy support, since most patients with depression seem to lack energy.

| Diabetes mellitus type 2 | 2 paraspinal MP level at T7–T9(B) attached to the paraspinal MP level with L2(B): EA Then separately TNP(B): EA | Attach the 2 thoracic paraspinal MP together with one lead and then clip the L2 paraspinal MP. Stay on the same side of the spine for this upper portion of the protocol. Repeat on the opposite side. Now you attach the right TNP (SP6) to the left TNP (SP6) with one lead. Both are plugged into the millicurrent settings. | EA: 2 HZ millicurrent for 30 minutes. 2–3 times week for 4 weeks. | This is a very effective protocol for instantly reducing high levels of blood sugar. I have used this and tested the patient's blood sugar for up to 3 hours after the treatment and have seen 90+ point reductions. When treating diabetes, keep in mind that diet, herbs, and stress management need to be addressed. |
| Diabetic neuropathy— lower leg | DPNP–CPNP: EA, TNP– SNP: EA | Use one lead to attach DPNP to CPNP, then use a second lead to attach SNP to TNP, all on the same leg. | EA: 25 HZ microcurrent for 25 minutes. 2 times a week for 6 weeks = 12 sessions. 3 times a week for 4 weeks = 12 sessions. | The microcurrent is what helps to heal the capillaries and repair the local soft tissue. You want the stimulation to be just noticeable in the beginning, and after several treatments work up to a comfortably strong sensation, but never a strong, uncomfortable feeling. It must be gentle. |

Disease/ condition	Neuropuncture acupoint prescription	EA placement explanation	Neuropuncture dosage	Commentary
Digestion/ constipation	SE25–ST36: EA	Use one lead to attach the right ST25 to the right ST36, then do the same on the opposite side.	EA: 10 HZ millicurrent for 20 minutes.	This protocol increases intestinal motility.
Energy/ fatigue (cellular respiration)	TNP(B): EA	In this simple but effective protocol, attach one lead to the right TNP, and the other to the left TNP, and EA.	EA: 2 HZ millicurrent for 25 minutes	This is excellent to combine light stimulation on a patient for insomnia while normal needling HT7, or in conjunction with other "Yin," hormone, or blood-deficient protocols.

Fatigue/ weakness/ deficiencies	ST36(B): EA, TNP(B): EA	Use one lead to attach ST36 to the opposite ST36. Then use a second lead to attach TNP (SP6) to the opposite TNP (SP6).	EA: 2 HZ millicurrent for 25 minutes.	This is a very simple and easy protocol, yet it is very effective. You should feel a marked difference in TCM pulse within 10 minutes. By the end of the treatment the pulses should be full, higher in level if it was originally deep, and much stronger than prior to treatment. If not, this indicates the severe nature of the deficiencies. (For a more specific immune system boost, see the Immune support protocol.) This protocol has been shown to help reduce oxidative stress in the body, especially the brain, and at 100 Hz has a neuroprotective effect on the brain.

Disease/ condition	Neuropuncture acupoint prescription	EA placement explanation	Neuropuncture dosage	Commentary
Herniated nucleus prolapse (HNP) with radiating pain	HTJJ C5–SRNP: EA	Attach one lead to the HTJJ points and the other lead to the distal neuropuncture point.	EA: 25 HZ microcurrent, for 25 minutes.	Cervical, C5, HNP with radiating pain into the thumb and index fingers.
	HTJJ C6–MNP: EA		EA: 25 HZ microcurrent, for 25 minutes.	Cervical, C6, HNP with radiating pain into the middle finger and palm.
	HTJJ L4/L5–CPNP: EA		EA: 25 HZ microcurrent, for 25 minutes.	Lumbar, L4/5, HNP with radiating pain into the leg and lateral aspect of calf.

| Herniated nucleus prolapse (HNP) with radiculopathy | C-spine/L-spine HNP: HTJJ level of HNP- Neuropuncture NP: EA | Here you use one lead to attach the HTJJ; if needling several HTJJs you should still use one alligator clip to grip them together, then connect to a distal Neuropuncture point on the affected neural pathway, using the same lead.

Your focus here is to target the pathological exiting nerve. So, for a C5 HNP, needle the HTJJ points level with C4/5/6 and attach them to SRNP and EA. | EA: Begin with 25 HZ microcurrent for 25 minutes. In subsequent sessions, increase to 2 HZ millicurrent, then to "mixed" stimulation at 2–15 HZ millicurrent, then to 2–100 HZ millicurrent. (See Chapter 5.) | Be sure to needle deep into the HTJJ points. It is okay if you tap the bone with the tip of the needle. Just use firm, gentle pressure when needling.

Always be careful of underlying anatomical structures, especially viscera. |

Disease/ condition	Neuropuncture acupoint prescription	EA placement explanation	Neuropuncture dosage	Commentary
Hypertension	MNP–PC5: EA, ST36–37(B): EA	Use one lead for each side and each protocol: • Use one lead to connect the right MNP (PC6) to PC5. • Use another lead to attach the left MNP (PC6) to PC5. • Use another lead to attach the right ST36 to the right ST37. • Attach the last lead to attach the left ST36 to the left ST37. All leads are inserted into the millicurrent plug-ins and switched to "mixed" frequency with the timer set for 30 minutes.	EA: 2–5 Hz millicurrent for 30 minutes. 2 times per week for 4–6 weeks.	I have seen this particular study (from UC, Irvine) twice recently. It is important to remember that diet, herbs, and stress management are also very important. What I like to do is treat a patient following a herbs, diet, and lifestyle regime, for 4–6 weeks, 2 times a week, and monitor.
Immune support	ST36(B): EA, REN4–DU20: EA	Use one lead to attach the right ST36 to the left ST36. Then use another lead to attach REN4 to DU20 (Pai Hui).	EA: 4 Hz millicurrent for 30 minutes.	Aside from the obvious immune-challenged patients who can benefit from this protocol, I also use it on patients undergoing chemotherapy. I treat them on the same day as they receive chemotherapy, and continue throughout their course of chemotherapy.

Infertility (dimished ovarian reserve)	Zi Gong Xue–TNP(B): EA	Use one lead to attach Zi Gong Xue to TNP on the same side. Repeat on the other side. When needling Zi Gong Xue, be sure to needle into the abdominal muscles. On thin patients use "serin blues."	EA: 2–15 HZ millicurrent for 12 weeks (5 times a week for 4 weeks, followed by 3 times a week for 8 weeks).	This has been shown to be effective for diminished ovarian reserve infertility.
Migraine/ headache	SRNP–GANP: EA, TNP– DPNP: EA	Here you use one lead to connect the right SRNP (LI4) to GANP, and then another lead to connect the left SRNP (LI4) to GANP. Use another lead to connect the right TNP (SP6) to DPNP (LV3), and the last lead to connect the left TNP (SP6) to DPNP (LV3). (Use 4 leads altogether.)	EA: 25 HZ microcurrent for 25 minutes. After 2 sessions, switch to 2 HZ millicurrent for the remainder of the sessions. 2 times a week for 4–6 weeks.	It is also a great idea to needle the HTJJ acupuncture points of the cervical spine and the Neuropuncture acupoints GOCNP/LOCNP/ TRAPMP. You can switch between protocols for the first week.

Disease/ condition	Neuropuncture acupoint prescription	EA placement explanation	Neuropuncture dosage	Commentary
Pain				
Chronic pain			Milli-stages of frequencies accordingly.	When it comes to pain there are several different approaches. Target a specific receptor with a specific frequency. Polarize a specific neural pathway. Interrupt pain signaling at a specific spinal segment.
Acute pain	Local ahshi points: EA through the injury.		EA: 25 HZ microcurrent to reduce inflammation and begin tissue repair.	
Knee pain	ST36–VMMP: EA, Xiyan-Dubi: EA With medial meniscus injuries, add LV8– SNP (SP9).	Use one lead to attach ST36 to vastus medialis motor point (VMMP), then another lead to attach Xiyan to Dubi.	EA: 2 HZ millicurrent. Begin with 2–3 treatments per week (1 week may suffice, depending on the condition).	

| Parkinson's disease | GB34–LV3(DPNP): EA
SP6(TNP)–ST36: EA | There is a simple self-explanatory protocol for Parkinson's disease. Simply use one lead to attach GB34 to LV3 on the same side. | SP6(TNP)–ST36: EA @ 100 HZ neuroprotective effect.
GB43–LV3(DPNP): EA @ 4 HZ tyrosine hydroxylase. All millicurrent. | The protocol has been shown to affect tyrosine hydroxylase and increase the production of dopamine.

Other research on long-term high-frequency EA shows that it not only halts the degeneration of dopaminergic neurons in the substantia nigra, but also upregulates the level of brain-derived neurotrophic factor (BNDF) mRNA in the subfields of the ventral midbrain, and stimulates the regeneration of the injured dopaminergic neurons (Jiang, 2009).

I like to combine this with the *Neuropuncture Alzheimer's/Dementia protocol* to add the neuroprotective properties. |

Disease/ condition	Neuropuncture acupoint prescription	EA placement explanation	Neuropuncture dosage	Commentary
Tinnitus/ hearing loss	SRNP–GANP: EA, TRIFNP– APNP: EA	Here you use one lead to attach SRNP to GANP, on the same side. Then use one lead to attach TRIFNP to APNP on the same side. Repeat on the other side if there are bi-lateral symptoms. This protocol runs current directly through the ear and along nerves that innervate the ear itself.	EA: 25 HZ microcurrent for 25 minutes. 2 times a week for 6 weeks = 12 sessions. 3 times a week for 4 weeks = 12 sessions.	This is a protocol that I designed myself to specifically target the neurology of the ear and tinnitus.

The idea is that by stimulating SRNP and GANP you are stimulating the cervical and brachial plexi together.

By stimulating the TRIFNP and ACNP you are running the microcurrent directly through the ear.

In combination it has a powerful effect on tinnitus and hearing loss. Again, though tinnitus is a tricky condition to treat, I have had some excellent results with this protocol. |

Chapter 9
Future Thoughts

I have read this over many times, and every time I continue to get excited about the applications of Neuropuncture and how many patients will be helped. This work is far from finished. I will continue to watch, research, and wonder how the new developments in neuroscience can be applied to acupuncture and its mechanisms. My current areas of research are the neuroscience of auricular mechanisms and protocols, scalp acupuncture systems and EA applied to the scalp, and the neurophysiological mechanisms for not only single but traditional acupuncture point prescriptions. There are many traditional acupuncture point prescriptions that have profound effects on modulating the nervous system, and the underlying mechanisms are still unclear. Another area of research is TCM pattern differential diagnosis associated with acupuncture point prescriptions and a comparison of the point prescription neurophysiological mechanisms with the Western pathology and pharmacokinetics of the medication of the disease being treated.

I will be further researching new Neuropuncture acupoints with their neuroanatomical mechanisms and conditions treated, as well as EA Neuropuncture acupoint protocols in the area of spinal cord nerve regeneration, stem cell proliferation, and oncology. I teach workshops that offer hands-on training in Neuropuncture, Neuropuncture certification programs, and short internship programs. Thank you—I hope that you enjoyed this book!

Respectfully,

Michael D. Corradino, DAOM, MTOM, L.AC.

References

Bensky, Dan, and John O'Connor. *Acupuncture: A Comprehensive Text.* Seattle: Eastland Press, 1991.

Bun, Hung Hung. *Dense Cranial Electroacupuncture Stimulation for Depression: Its Clinical Efficacy and Neuroimaging Evidence from Randomized Controlled Studies.* PhD thesis. Hong Kong: University of Hong Kong, 2014.

Cheng, N, H Van Hoof, E Bockx, MJ Hoogmartens *et al.* "The effects of electric currents on ATP generation, protein synthesis, and membrane transport of rat skin." *Clinical Orthopaedics and Related Research*, Vol 171, Nov–Dec 1982, pp.264–272.

Cheng, Xinnong, and Liangyue Deng. *Chinese Acupuncture and Moxibustion.* Beijing: Foreign Languages Press, 1999.

Fernandes, CA, YK Nóbrega, and CE Tosta. "Pranic meditation affects phagocyte functions and hormonal levels of recent practitioners." *Journal of Alternative and Complementary Medicine*, Vol 18, Number 8, 2012, pp.761–768.

Filshie, Jacqueline, and Adrian White. *Medical Acupuncture: A Western Scientific Approach.* New York: Churchill Livingstone, 1998.

Frisaldi, E, A Piedimonte, and F Benedetti. "Placebo and nocebo effects: a complex interplay between psychological factors and neurochemical networks." *American Journal of Clinical Hypnosis*, Vol 57, Number 3, 2015, pp.267–284.

Golianau, Brenda, MD, and Elizabeth Sebestyen, MD. *Does Electro-Acupuncture Potentiate Chemotherapy in Cancer Patients?* 3rd International Medical Congress on Acupuncture, Barcelona, 2007.

Hindrichs, TJ, and LL Barnes. *Chinese Medicine and Healing.* Cambridge, Mass: Harvard University Press, 2013.

Jiang, Y, MD, PhD. "Acupuncture in the treatment of Parkinson's disease." *North American Journal of Medical Science*, Vol 2, Number 1, 2009, pp.32–34.

Jing-Nuan, Wu. *Ling Shu or The Spiritual Pivot.* Hawaii: University of Hawaii Press, 1993.

Maciocia, Giovanni. *The Foundations of Chinese Medicine: A Comprehensive Text for Acupuncturists and Herbalists.* Edinburgh, London, Melbourne, and New York: Churchill Livingstone, 1989.

Mann, F. *Reinventing Acupuncture: A New Concept of Ancient Medicine.* Oxford: Butterworth Heinemann, 2000.

Marieb, Elaine N, and Katja Hoehn. *Human Anatomy and Physiology.* San Francisco: Benjamin Cummings, 2009.

Pokorny, J. "Biophysical aspects of cancer – electromagnetic mechanism." *Indian Journal of Experimental Biology*, Vol. 46, May 2008, pp.310–321.

Rohen, Johannes W, Chirhiro Yokochi, and Elke Lutjen-Drecoll. *Color Atlas of Anatomy: A Photographic Study of the Human Body (Fifth Edition).* Philadelphia: Lippincott Williams and Wilkins, 2003.

Unshuld, Paul U. *Nan-Ching: The Classic of Difficult Issues.* Los Angeles: University of California Press, 1986.

Wang, Zhao, and Jun Wang. *Ling Shu Acupuncture.* Anaheim: Ling Shu Press, 2007.

White, A, and J Campbell. "Acupuncture is rational medicine." *British Medical Journal Online*, 24 May 2005, www.bmj.com/rapid-response/2011/10/30/acupuncture-rational-medicine.

White, Adrian, Mike Cummings, and Jacqueline Filshie. *An Introduction to Western Medical Acupuncture.* London: Elsevier Health Sciences, 2008.

Index

brain *cont.*
  limbic area 28
  neuroanatomy 25–36, *37*
  primitive 28
  subcortex 59
  tumors of 73
brainstem 57, 73
burns 48

calcitonin gene-related peptide (CGRP) 34,
    40–1, 49, 60
cancer, electrochemotherapy for 72–4
carpal tunnel release Neuropuncture
    acupoint/nerves 106, *107*
central nervous system (CNS) 26, 27, 41
  chemical dependency 58–9
  depression 60
  Electro-Acupuncture (EA) as physical
      therapy for 63
  endocrinology 59–60
  immunology 58
  mechanism 58–60
  nausea and vomiting 60
  oxytocin 60
  stimulating via millicurrent/microcurrent
      71–2
central pain 44
cerebral cortex 25, 27–8, 29
cervical column 55
cervical plexus 30
C-fibers 30, 33, 40, 51
CGRP (calcitonin gene-related peptide) 34,
    40–1, 49, 60
chemical dependency 58–9
chemical soup 23, 49, 50, 61
China 59
cholesterol, brain 27
chronic pain 46–7
cingulate gyrus 25, 29
CNS see central nervous system (CNS)
common peroneal Neuropuncture
    acupoint/nerves 112, 113
cortex, brain 25, 27–8, 29, 41, 59
current, Electro-Acupuncture 63–4
cytokines 40, 44

De Qi sensation 22, *24*, 33, 77
  comfortable 51, 52, 74, 134, 135, 136
  Electro-Acupuncture (EA) 142
  obtaining locally 50–1
deep cranial Electro-Acupuncture (DCEA) 71
deep median Neuropuncture acupoint/
    nerves 102, 103
deep peroneal Neuropuncture acupoint/
    nerves 118, 119
deep radial acupoint/nerves 98, 99
delta fibers 19
delta receptor 32, 56
dendrites 31
depolarization, nerves 31
depression 60
dermatomes 36
Descartes, R. 39, 40
descending pain system 31, 57
diffuse intrinsic pontine plioma (DIPG) 73
docosahexaenoic acid (DHA) molecules 32
dorsal horn 41, 53, 54, 55, 57, 72
Dunn, James 69
Duong Ha (Dr.) 70
dynorphin 32, 56

EA see Electro-Acupuncture (EA)
efferent nerve fibers 33
Electro-Neuropuncture (EN) 136–8
  protocols 142–3
Electro-Acupuncture (EA) 27–8, 41, 62–74
  all or none theory 31
  auricular Electro-Acupuncture (EA) 47, 59
  bi-phasic wave patterns 65
  clinical settings 67–8
  contraindications 74
  current 63–4
  Kelly Protocol 75, *76*
  machine types 65, 143
  neural synapse *66*
  pain treatment 67–8
  as physical therapy for CNS 63
  theories 68–72
  treatment protocols 141
  see also acupuncture
electrochemotherapy 72–4